Fitness & Health

Series Editor: Cara Acred

Volume 313

WITHDRAWN

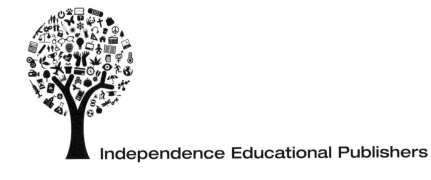

Independence Educational Publishers

First published by Independence Educational Publishers

The Studio, High Green

Great Shelford

Cambridge CB22 5EG

England

© Independence 2017

ISBN-13: 978 1 86168 763 0

Printed in Great Britain

Zenith Print Group

Contents

Introduction

FITNESS & HEALTH is Volume 313 in the **ISSUES** series. The aim of the series is to offer current, diverse information about important issues in our world, from a UK perspective.

ABOUT FITNESS & HEALTH

With increasing advancements in fitness-tracking technology, it is easier than ever to monitor our day-to-day activity levels. But just how much activity should we be doing? And why do so many of us still fall short? This book looks at the topic of fitness, exploring issues such as HIIT workouts and children's health. It also considers how fitness relates to the obesity epidemic that is sweeping the globe and presents potential solutions.

OUR SOURCES

Titles in the **ISSUES** series are designed to function as educational resource books, providing a balanced overview of a specific subject.

The information in our books is comprised of facts, articles and opinions from many different sources, including:

⇨ Newspaper reports and opinion pieces

⇨ Website factsheets

⇨ Magazine and journal articles

⇨ Statistics and surveys

⇨ Government reports

⇨ Literature from special interest groups.

A NOTE ON CRITICAL EVALUATION

Because the information reprinted here is from a number of different sources, readers should bear in mind the origin of the text and whether the source is likely to have a particular bias when presenting information (or when conducting their research). It is hoped that, as you read about the many aspects of the issues explored in this book, you will critically evaluate the information presented.

It is important that you decide whether you are being presented with facts or opinions. Does the writer give a biased or unbiased report? If an opinion is being expressed, do you agree with the writer? Is there potential bias to the 'facts' or statistics behind an article?

ASSIGNMENTS

In the back of this book, you will find a selection of assignments designed to help you engage with the articles you have been reading and to explore your own opinions. Some tasks will take longer than others and there is a mixture of design, writing and research-based activities that you can complete alone or in a group.

Useful weblinks

www.bupa.co.uk

www.cancerresearchuk.org

www.theconversation.com

www.diabetes.co.uk

www.esrc.ac.uk

www.europeanobesityday.eu

www.exeter.ac.uk

www.fieldsintrust.org

www.fitforsport.co.uk

www.fullfact.org

GOV.uk

www.theguardian.com

www.huffingtonpost.co.uk

www.independent.co.uk

www.local.gov.uk

www.mind.org.uk

www.mobilenewscwp.co.uk

www.nhs.uk

www.nuffieldfoundation.org

www.parliament.uk

www.telegraph.co.uk

www.ukactive.com

www.worldobesity.org

www.yougov.co.uk

FURTHER RESEARCH

At the end of each article we have listed its source and a website that you can visit if you would like to conduct your own research. Please remember to critically evaluate any sources that you consult and consider whether the information you are viewing is accurate and unbiased.

Exercise – getting started

A quick poll around our office showed that "feeling too tired" and "not having enough time" were among the main things stopping people from exercising. And yet in a survey for 'Feel Great Britain' both "doing something active outdoors" and "exercising" made it into the top 50 things that make people feel great.

So really we should all be getting active – and it may be easier than you think. Here we give you tips and advice for getting started.

How much exercise should I do?

The UK Department of Health has set down minimum recommendations for how much exercise different age groups should aim to do. Don't be put off if these seem a lot. If you're just getting started, go slow at first and gradually increase the amount and intensity of activity you do to build up your fitness. Trying to do too much too quickly may mean you lose motivation and stop. Adding just five minutes will help you reach your target and increase your fitness levels.

To get all the benefits of exercise, each week adults should aim to do:

⇨   at least two and a half hours of moderate intensity exercise over a week in bouts of ten minutes or more

OR

⇨   an hour and 15 minutes of vigorous intensity activity

OR

⇨   an equal mix of moderate and vigorous intensity activity

AND

⇨   at least twice-weekly activities that build up muscle strength, such as lifting weights or exercises using your body weight (push-ups and sit-ups for example).

Moderate intensity means:

⇨   your breathing is faster

⇨   your heart rate is faster

⇨   you feel warmer.

Vigorous intensity means:

⇨   your breathing is much deeper and more rapid

⇨   your heart rate increases quickly.

Weekly exercise plans

There are plenty of ways to pack activity into your week so you'll probably reach the target before you know it. Here are some sample exercise routines to achieve them:

Exercise	How long?	How often?
Walking (brisk)	30 minutes	5 times a week
Walking (brisk)	15 minutes	2 times a day, 5 days a week
Running	25 minutes	3 times a week
Skipping	15 minutes	6 times a week
Walking… and running	30 minutes 30 minutes	2 times a week 2 times a week
Cycling (with few hills)… and swimming (fast)	30 minutes 30 minutes	2 times a week 2 times a week

"I've joined a running club that I go to once a week. I was a bit wary at first as I'm a total beginner but they were so welcoming and I've really surprised myself with what I've achieved. I won't be doing a marathon any time soon but I've signed up to do a 5km race with some friends from the club."

Becca, doctor

Set goals for exercise

It's a good idea to set some goals when you start exercising. Think about what you're aiming to get out of the effort you're going to be putting in. Making your goals 'SMART' can help you.

⇨   **Specific** – say exactly what you will do. For example, you'll go to the gym twice a week before work.

⇨   **Measurable** – if you can't measure your goal, you won't know if you've achieved it. If you ride a bike, time how long it takes to cycle a set distance and keep track of how this improves.

⇨   **Attainable** – your goal needs to be something you can and are willing to do. Although "I'll run a marathon by my next birthday" is admirable, if you've not run before and don't enjoy it, it's unlikely to happen. Why not sign up to a 5km in three months' time instead.

⇨   **Realistic** – something you can do with the resources you have. Although it might be nice to have a personal

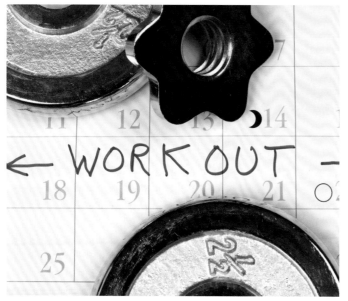

trainer, perhaps a group exercise class is more in line with your finances.

⇨ **Time-based** – give yourself a sensible time frame in which to meet your goal. An example might be to be able to swim a mile after a month of regular swimming sessions.

Having goals is also great for reminding yourself how much you've improved and tracking your progress – think how great you'll feel if just a few months after you start jogging, you can complete a 5km run.

Make exercise fun

If the thought of exercise fills you with dread, choose an activity you enjoy. You don't have to go to the gym to get the health benefits of exercise.

If running puts you off, try an aerobics or dance class instead. Or perhaps yoga or tai chi is more your style? Have a go at a few things until you find some that suit you.

We've put together some of our favourites to give you ideas – both moderate and vigorous intensity depending on how energetic you're feeling (see table below)

Once you've chosen an exercise you enjoy, you need to stay motivated and stick with it. The following may help.

⇨ Put your goal on paper and stick it on the fridge so you have a constant reminder of what you're aiming to achieve.

⇨ Use mobile phone apps to measure your progress. Structured exercise plans as well as personal trainer apps are freely available. If walking is your thing, download our Ground Miles app and walk your way to health and well being.

⇨ Maybe you find it helps if you have a plan to follow. We have a range of running training programmes for different distances – if you're just starting out, try our walking programme or 'walk to run' 5km plan.

⇨ Bring out your competitive spirit. Enter yourself into a charity run so you have something to aim for, or join a sports league that has regular fixtures.

Build exercise into your life

You're likely to find it easier to do physical activity if you build it into your everyday life. Try to spend as little time as possible being inactive. You can include daily activities, structured exercise and sport, or a combination of these, into your weekly goal. It all counts. Here's just a selection of ideas to break down those barriers and get you more active without realising it.

Moderate intensity	*Vigorous intensity*
Take a bike ride with the family.	Head to a martial arts class.
Go for a brisk walk – make it more interesting by listening to some new music or a podcast while you walk.	Go for a run.
Go rollerblading – perfect for parks and proms.	Swimming, but really go for it – try racing with your kids.
Aquarobics is a good activity for everybody as the water supports your weight.	Aerobics will get your blood flowing.
Volleyball – it's a great team sport.	Hockey – this can be a great social opportunity.
Skateboarding – go on a downhill ride!	Cycling up hills – to keep going, think of the sense of achievement you'll have once you reach the top!
Gardening – make your outdoor spaces look enticing.	Basketball – you could sign up to a league.
Head out for a day hiking in the country.	Football – another great social sport.
Cleaning, such as vacuuming – it all counts!	Shovelling or carrying heavy loads – get your jobs done and a good workout at the same time.
Go dancing – it doesn't have to be a formal class, put some music on and dance around the living room.	Train for a stand up paddle (SUP) race – the latest watersport that's fun for all the family.
Play rounders in the park.	Try trapfit – the new exercise trend that's come over from the US where you exercise using a trapeze!
Take on your friends in doubles tennis.	Try piloxing, a combination of Pilates and boxing.

- If you have children and they take up the majority of your time, why not exercise with them? You could go on a family bike ride for example, or go bowling or ice-skating.

- If you have a busy work life, fit exercise around it. Head out early and hit the gym before work or wind down with a swim afterwards. It can be a great way to process the day.

- Walk or cycle to work or your kids to school a couple of days or more a week.

- Instead of watching TV in the evening, walk to and from the cinema to watch a film.

- Make the most of even small opportunities to be active – use the stairs, do manual tasks.

- Walk instead of driving short journeys, or get off the bus one or two stops earlier than usual.

- Build some activities into your weekend – do some DIY or gardening.

- Join an organised bike ride, running club or walking group. Knowing you have a commitment to do something with other people can be a great motivator.

One-week exercise plan

If you're still thinking you can't possibly fit activity into your lifestyle, you might be surprised by what you can achieve. Just see how easy it can be in an average week for a working person who commutes to the office. This example shows you can smash the target, just in everyday life!

Day	Activity	Time
Monday	Walk to the station and back; step out of the office to get some lunch	20 minutes / 10 minutes
Tuesday	Walk to the station and back; nip to the dry cleaners after work	20 minutes / 15 minutes
Wednesday	Walk to the station and back; go to a yoga class after work	20 minutes / 40 minutes
Thursday	Walk to the station and back	20 minutes
Friday		
Saturday	Vacuum the house	30 minutes
Sunday	Go for bike ride	60 minutes
Total		235 minutes

"I'm a freelancer so make sure I get out of the house at least once a day for a brisk walk with friends who also work from home. It's valuable contact with others and having a dog that demands walking helps!"

Rachael, freelance editor

What if I have a health condition?

A number of health conditions, such as osteoarthritis and back pain, may mean you feel anxious about exercising. But actually it's usually recommended that you keep active to help treat your symptoms. This might be with strengthening exercises or something more lively that gets your heart rate up. Both of these are thought to be better than bed rest or steering clear of activity.

Walking is very safe but if you have specific concerns, contact your GP about what you can and can't do. Or if you've been referred to another doctor or physiotherapist, they can recommend the activities and exercise that are most suitable for you.

Resources

Further information

British Heart Foundation National Centre for Physical Activity and Health
01509 226 421
www.bhfactive.org.uk

Sources

The 50 things that put the 'feel great' in Great Britain. Bupa. www.bupa.com, published 15 April 2015

Physical activity guidelines for adults (19–64 years) Department of Health. www.gov.uk, published July 2011

Moderate to vigorous – what is your level of intensity? American Heart Association. www.heart.org, published March 2014

Examples of moderate and vigorous physical activity. Harvard TH Chan School of Public Health. www.hsph.harvard.edu, accessed 11 June 2015

Measuring physical activity intensity. Centers for Disease Control and Prevention. www.cdc.gov, published 4 February 2015

Accessed 27 October 2016

- The above information is reprinted with kind permission from Bupa. Please visit www.bupa.co.uk for further information.

Benefits of exercise

Step right up! It's the miracle cure we've all been waiting for.

It can reduce your risk of major illnesses, such as heart disease, stroke, type 2 diabetes and cancer by up to 50% and lower your risk of early death by up to 30%.

It's free, easy to take, has an immediate effect and you don't need a GP to get some. Its name? Exercise.

Exercise is the miracle cure we've always had, but for too long we've neglected to take our recommended dose. Our health is now suffering as a consequence.

This is no snake oil. Whatever your age, there's strong scientific evidence that being physically active can help you lead a healthier and even happier life.

People who do regular activity have a lower risk of many chronic diseases, such as heart disease, type 2 diabetes, stroke, and some cancers.

Research shows that physical activity can also boost self-esteem, mood, sleep quality and energy, as well as reducing your risk of stress, depression, dementia and Alzheimer's disease.

"If exercise were a pill, it would be one of the most cost-effective drugs ever invented," says Dr Nick Cavill, a health promotion consultant.

Health benefits

Given the overwhelming evidence, it seems obvious that we should all be physically active. It's essential if you want to live a healthy and fulfilling life into old age.

It's medically proven that people who do regular physical activity have:

⇨ up to a 35% lower risk of coronary heart disease and stroke

⇨ up to a 50% lower risk of type 2 diabetes

⇨ up to a 50% lower risk of colon cancer

⇨ up to a 20% lower risk of breast cancer

⇨ a 30% lower risk of early death

⇨ up to an 83% lower risk of osteoarthritis

⇨ up to a 68% lower risk of hip fracture

⇨ a 30% lower risk of falls (among older adults)

⇨ up to a 30% lower risk of depression

⇨ up to a 30% lower risk of dementia.

What counts?

To stay healthy, adults should try to be active daily and aim to achieve at least 150 minutes of physical activity over a week through a variety of activities.

For most people, the easiest way to get moving is to make activity part of everyday life, like walking or cycling instead of using the car to get around. However, the more you do, the better, and taking part in activities such as sports and exercise will make you even healthier.

For any type of activity to benefit your health, you need to be moving quick enough to raise your heart rate, breathe faster and feel warmer. This level of effort is called moderate intensity activity. One way to tell if you're working at a moderate intensity is if you can still talk but you can't sing the words to a song.

If your activity requires you to work even harder, it is called vigorous intensity activity. There is substantial evidence that vigorous activity can bring health benefits over and above that of moderate activity. You can tell when it's vigorous activity because you're breathing hard and fast, and your heart rate has gone up quite a bit. If you're working at this level, you won't be able to say more than a few words without pausing for a breath.

A modern problem

People are less active nowadays, partly because technology has made our lives easier. We drive cars or take public transport. Machines wash our clothes. We entertain ourselves in front of a TV or computer screen. Fewer people are doing manual work, and most of us have jobs that involve little physical effort. Work, house chores, shopping and other necessary activities are far less demanding than for previous generations.

We move around less and burn off less energy than people used to. Research suggests that many adults spend more than seven hours a day sitting down, at work, on transport or in their leisure time. People aged over 65 spend ten hours or more each day sitting or lying down, making them the most sedentary age group.

Sedentary lifestyles

Inactivity is described by the Department of Health as a "silent killer". Evidence is emerging that sedentary behaviour, such as sitting or lying down for long periods, is bad for your health.

Not only should you try to raise your activity levels, but you should also reduce the amount of time you and your family spend sitting down.

Common examples of sedentary behaviour include watching TV, using a computer, using the car for short journeys and sitting down to read, talk or listen to music – and such behaviour is thought to increase your risk of many chronic diseases, such as heart disease, stroke and type 2 diabetes, as well as weight gain and obesity.

"Previous generations were active more naturally through work and manual labour, but today we have to find ways of integrating activity into our daily lives," says Dr Cavill.

Whether it's limiting the time babies spend strapped in their buggies, or encouraging adults to stand up and move frequently, people of all ages need to reduce their sedentary behaviour.

"This means that each of us needs to think about increasing the types of activities that suit our lifestyle and can easily be included in our day," says Dr Cavill.

Crucially, you can hit your weekly activity target but still be at risk of ill health if you spend the rest of the time sitting or lying down. For tips on building physical activity and exercise into your day, whatever your age, read *Get active your way* on the NHS Choices website.

13 July 2015

⇨ The above information is reprinted with kind permission from NHS Choices. Please visit www.nhs.uk for further information.

How physical activity prevents cancer

Being physically active isn't just good for your heart: there is lots of evidence that it can also reduce the risk of developing breast, bowel or womb cancer. Keeping active could help to prevent around 3,400 cases of cancer every year in the UK.

How does physical activity affect hormone levels?

Hormones are chemical messages that get carried around our bodies in our blood. They help tell our bodies and cells what to do. Being physically active can change the levels of some hormones, including oestrogen and insulin.

In women, physical activity can lower the level of oestrogen. Oestrogen is thought to fuel the development of many breast and womb cancers, so reducing the levels of this hormone could help to reduce the risk.

Activity can also reduce the amount of insulin in our blood. Insulin is very important in controlling how our bodies use and store energy from food. Changes in insulin levels can have effects all over the body. And scientists think insulin can turn on signals that tell cells to multiply. Because cancer starts when cells multiply out of control, lowering insulin levels could help stop some types of cancer from developing.

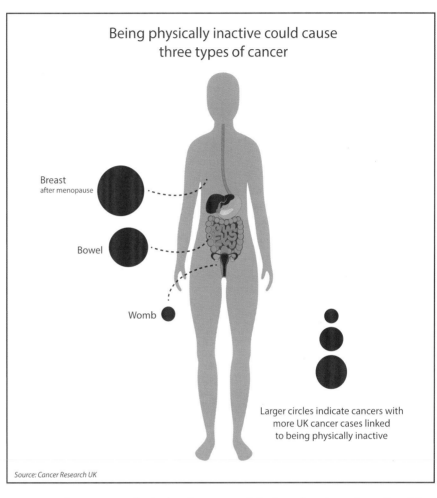

Being physically inactive could cause three types of cancer

Breast after menopause

Bowel

Womb

Larger circles indicate cancers with more UK cancer cases linked to being physically inactive

Source: Cancer Research UK

How does physical activity prevent bowel cancer?

Physical activity helps food move through our bowels. When food moves through our bowels quickly this reduces the amount of time that the inside lining of the bowel is in contact with any harmful chemicals, like those released when you consume alcohol or red and processed meat. So there's less chance of them being able to cause damage that could lead to cancer.

Being active also helps control levels of inflammation in the bowel. Inflammation is a normal part of the way our bodies react to injury or infections. But it can sometimes cause even more damage, particularly when it keeps happening in the same place. This can lead to the cells multiplying much more frequently than usual, to replace dead and damaged cells, increasing the chances of mistakes that could lead to cancer.

Is physical activity just good for us because of its effects on weight?

Being physically active, along with a healthy, balanced diet, can also help you manage your weight. And keeping to a healthy weight is another great way to reduce the risk of developing cancer and other diseases.

But physical activity has benefits above and beyond weight control, and it doesn't only reduce the risk of cancer through its effects on weight.

How does physical activity benefit cancer patients?

There is also good evidence that being active can help people during and following cancer treatment. If you are a cancer patient and want to be more active, discuss with your doctor what would work best for you.

24 March 2015

⇨ The above information is reprinted with kind permission from Cancer Research. Please visit www.cancerresearchuk.org for further information.

© Cancer Research UK 2017

What exercise does to your bones

An article from **The Conversation.**

By Alex Ireland, Postdoctoral Researcher in Neuromuscular and Skeletal Physiology, Manchester Metropolitan University

When we think of bones, a lifeless skeleton usually comes to mind, but our bones are a living organ that grows and changes shape throughout our life. Much of this shaping results from forces which press, pull and twist the skeleton as we move, and the biggest of these forces is caused by our muscles.

Bones experience huge forces during movement. When a triple jumper's heel hits the ground, the force is around 15 times their body weight – or the weight of a small car. In fact, because muscles normally attach close to joints, muscular forces are even greater than these impact forces (in the same way that you have to push harder to lift someone on a see-saw the closer you get to the middle). As a result bones also experience huge impact and muscle force during daily tasks, totalling more than five times body weight even during walking.

These forces squash, twist and bend bones. The shin bone briefly becomes nearly a millimetre shorter as your foot hits the ground when running. The bone senses these small changes, and can grow dramatically – in the months after starting exercise – in order to reduce the risk of breaking. For example, the racket arm bones of tennis players can be 20% wider and contain 40% more bone mineral than their other arm, while sprint runners have up to a third more bone in their shin bone than people who don't exercise.

But not all exercise gives us big, strong bones. We seem to need high impacts (hitting the floor from a jump, or striking a tennis ball) to produce big enough muscle and impact forces to make our bones change. As a result, not all exercise appears to be beneficial for bone. Swimmers and cyclists may have healthy hearts, lungs and muscles but their bones are not much different from people who do not exercise.

Bone's response to these forces varies along its length. Near the joints, bones get bigger and more dense, whereas bone shafts tend to get bigger and thicker with little change in bone density. Bones also change in shape. The shin bone shaft starts as a circular tube, but gets wider from front to back as we grow and start to move until it forms a tear-drop shape. But if we start to load our bones less, they waste away and these effects are no less dramatic. Astronauts lose up to 1% of their leg bone mass per month when in space, while people who suffer a spinal cord injury lose up to half of their shin bone mass.

Stronger bones for life

This shaping of bones by forces appears to occur throughout life. Even at 15 months old, children who started to walk early have up to 40% more bone in their shin than children who have yet to start walking; effects that last until at least their late teens. Bone seems to be most sensitive to loading while we're still growing. Once we reach our final height, bone appears less able to increase its width, particularly near the joints. While some of the benefits gradually disappear once you stop exercising, exercised bones remain wider even several decades after exercise stops.

This suggests that exercise in childhood may give us bigger, stronger bones for life. This is important as bigger, stronger bones are less likely to break as we get older. Certainly, exercise trials can be very effective in making children's bones stronger, and also in reducing bone loss from bed rest or even partly reversing bone loss in spinal cord injury.

However, effects of exercise on bone in elderly people have so far been much smaller. This is a big problem as we break our bones more often as we get older. The lack of large improvements in bone quality as a result of exercise in older people might be because we can't produce as much force as we get older, or that bones are less sensitive to the forces we do produce. Alternatively, it could be that changes in our muscles and bones mean that the amount of squashing, bending and twisting our bones experiences during movement also changes. New techniques allow us to look at these patterns for the first time, which should allow us to plan more effective exercises in people of all ages.

Forces acting on our bones during everyday movements and exercise have a strong influence on the size, shape and strength of our bones. If we move less this can make our bones weak and more likely to break, but being active and doing exercise such as running, football or tennis can help make our bones much stronger. At the moment, exercise trials seem most effective in children and in stopping or slowing bone loss in disuse. However, ongoing work is giving us a much clearer picture of how forces contort our bones during different movements. This will allow us to design more effective exercises for bone in different groups, finally allowing us to translate the dramatic effects of exercise on bone seen in athletes into benefits for the wider population.

20 April 2016

⇨ The above information is reprinted with kind permission from *The Conversation*. Please visit www.theconversation.com for further information.

High intensity exercise could cause an abnormal heart beat, sports cardiologist suggests

Fitness fanatics who overdo it at the gym could be more likely to suffer from an abnormal heart rhythm, an independent review has suggested.

The sports cardiologist behind the review, Dr André La Gerche, believes that high levels of intense exercise are "cardiotoxic" and could increase the likelihood of suffering permanent structural changes in the heart, leading to arrhythmias (an abnormal heart beat).

He said that it is important to do exercise to stay healthy. But added that there is compelling evidence supporting the association between carrying out long-term high intensity training and the development of heart problems.

Sports cardiologist Dr André La Gerche, head of sports cardiology at the Baker IDI Heart and Diabetes Institute in Australia, said that the question of whether too much exercise is bad for a person's health is often "hijacked by definitive media-grabbing statements".

This, he said, has "fuelled" an environment in which a person might be criticised for even questioning the benefits of exercise.

"This paper discusses the often questionable, incomplete, and controversial science behind the emerging concern that high levels of intense exercise may be associated with some adverse health effects," he said.

Dr Gerche's review looked at existing data surrounding high intensity exercise and how it could cause adverse cardiac changes in some athletes.

He said that all therapies – whether that's medication or fitness – have a "dose-response relationship". In other words, if you take too many pills or complete too much exercise, it has a negative impact on health.

According to Dr Gerche, there is a commonly held view that heart problems which develop in athletes are often blamed on an underlying abnormality, which is then triggered by exercise.

But he believes that exercise could actually be the cause for these issues.

In his study, he questioned whether there was a "non-linear dose-response relationship with exercise" and whether "endurance exercise in athletes was associated with arrhythmias".

He said that there was a lot of conflicting evidence between studies, especially as larger population studies supporting the health benefits of exercise often dwarfed smaller cross-sectional studies that examined whether intense exercise could be bad for health.

"The answers regarding the healthfulness of 'extreme' exercise are not complete and there are valid questions being raised," he said in his review.

"Given that this is a concern that affects such a large proportion of society, it is something that deserves investment.

"The lack of large prospective studies of persons engaged in high-volume and high-intensity exercise represents the biggest deficiency in the literature to date, and, although such work presents a logistical and financial challenge, many questions will remain controversies until such data emerge."

He said further investigation, with large-scale studies, is needed to establish the effect of intense exercise on heart structure and function.

The review was published in the *Canadian Journal of Cardiology*.

26 February 2016

⇨ The above information is reprinted with kind permission from The Huffington Post UK. Please visit www.huffingtonpost.co.uk for further information.

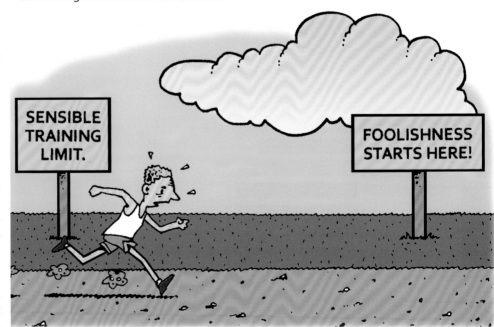

Brits missing NHS exercise targets, with women aged 40–54 the worst offenders

In conjunction with Simply Health, YouGov has launched an everyday health tracker, with the aim of painting the broadest picture yet of UK health and wellbeing.

By Ben Tobin

One major finding the first wave of research has unearthed is that UK adults are falling well below NHS exercise targets, with only a minority meeting current recommendations on aerobic activity.

"31% say that they are aware of the NHS aerobic activity target, but only 40% assert that they met the target over the last three months"

The NHS aerobic activity target is 150 minutes moderate intensity per week (e.g. fast walking/cycling) or 75 minutes vigorous intensity per week (e.g. running, tennis).

31% say that they are aware of the NHS aerobic activity target, but only 40% assert that they met the target over the last three months. 39% are doing less than one session per week. Only one in seven (14%) know about the muscle-strengthening activity target.

Women perform worse than men on this front, and this is true across all age groups. Women aged 40–54 are the least likely to exercise the recommended amount, just 32% do. 25–39 year old men are most likely to (51%).

What explains the disparity between the recommendation and the reality? Almost one third (32%) say the lack of time is the reason, while the same number say it is lack of willpower to blame.

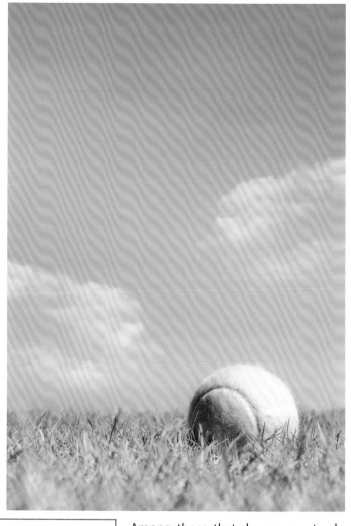

Everyday health tracker
Frequency of 30 minute sessions of aerobic activity over the last three months

Frequency	Percentage
At least once a day	9%
Six times a week	3%
Five times a week	6%
Four times a week	9%
Three times a week	13%
Two times a week	11%
Once a week	11%
Once every two weeks	5%
Once every month	5%
Less often	29%

Source: YouGov, 2015

Among those that do manage to do regular aerobic exercise, the most popular reason for doing it is simply "to feel better overall" (50%). 47% want to raise the general fitness while 41% say their motivation is to lose weight. Other reasons include "to increase energy levels" (20%) and increase attractiveness to others (8%).

13 August 2015

⇨ The above information is reprinted with kind permission from YouGov Please visit www.yougov.co.uk for further information.

© YouGov 2017

School PE nightmares mean women shun exercise – putting them at risk of poor physical and mental health

Women with mental health problems are not exercising because of bad experiences with PE at school – putting them at greater risk of poor physical, and mental, health the charity Mind has warned. More than half of women (57%) do not participate in sport because they were not good at PE at school[1] while nearly half (43%) feel it is too competitive.

In response, Mind has launched a new motivational website to help women with mental health problems choose a sport which is suitable for them, enabling them to take the first step and get active to improve their physical and mental well being.

Women with mental health problems are more likely to have physical health problems such as diabetes and heart disease so being active can be really important for looking after their physical health. Mind's new website is part of the charity's physical activity project, Get Set to Go, supported by Sport England and the National Lottery.

Mind's new website asks people to select reasons stopping them from exercising, and provides practical tips and real-life stories to inspire people to take the first step, and reap the benefits of an active lifestyle.

22-year-old Louise from London was diagnosed with Generalised Anxiety Disorder in her second year of university. She started running with help from Couch to 5k after her GP encouraged her to try exercise and has found that running helps her to manage her mental health.

"I've found that running has made a real difference to how I cope with my anxiety. I was very unwell last July after I finished university but running makes me feel in control of the monsters in my brain. As well as giving me more energy and increasing my fitness, being active has made me appreciate my body.

"Running was a battle with my mind, more than my body, which is true for runners with or without mental health problems. But I'm glad that I pushed through the negative thoughts telling me to stop running as I'm so much more positive now. And fitter!"

Women currently exercise less often than men,[2] but want to do more physical activity,[3] so Mind is calling on women to use the charity's new website to help them break down the common barriers – including feeling worried about taking part by themselves and fear of crowded spaces – which stop them from getting started.

Hayley Jarvis, Community Programmes Manager (Sport) at Mind, says: "We know that having a mental health problem can make getting active more difficult. The thought of joining a running group when you have bipolar disorder, depression or OCD can stop you in your tracks – but a mental health problem doesn't have to prevent anybody from getting active. Our new website is full of practical tips and inspirational real life stories which can help people take the first step, and reap the benefits of an active lifestyle.

"Being active can be an enjoyable, fun and social way of looking after your physical and mental health. Lots of people tell us it is a great way to socialise and make new friends – and there is a huge number of activities people can do if they struggle with social situations or new faces," Hayley adds.

Last summer Mind released findings which showed that 85% of women with mental health problems did not participate in sport because they don't feel confident in their sporting ability. More than half (56%) told the charity they are not "gym body ready", saying they are not members of sports clubs, gyms or leisure centres, because they are embarrassed about their body shape or size.

Through Get Set to Go, Mind aims to support 75,000 people with mental health problems to improve their lives through physical activity. The programme supports people with mental health problems become more active through eight sports projects across England. Those taking part receive one-to-one support from others with shared experiences, who understand the additional challenges a mental health problem presents to those who want to get active. Participants also get support through Mind's safe and supportive online social network Elefriends, by swapping tips, advice and linking up with others who are just starting out.

For more information, to find out about projects in your area and to use Mind's new website, visit www.mind.org.uk/sport. To talk to other people about getting started with sport visit Mind's social network Elefriends, www.elefriends.org.uk.

References

1. Mind conducted a Survey Monkey poll of 660 people (488 of whom have mental health problems) between 11 May and 6 July 2015.

2. Sport England: Active People Survey 9 (1.73 million more men played sport once a week compared to women).

3. Sport England: Go where women are (13 million women say they would like to participate more in sport and physical activity – just over six million of those women are not currently active).

11 April 2016

⇨ The above information is reprinted with kind permission from Mind. Please visit www.mind.org.uk for further information.

Not just child's play – study provides benchmark for identifying those at risk

Boys perform better than girls in speed, limb strength and cardiorespiratory fitness, whilst girls have the edge in balance and flexibility, according to a landmark study of European children which hopes to provide useful data in the fight against childhood obesity and other health issues.

Over 10,000 children aged between six and 11 took part in the research, which is the first to provide sex and age-specific physical reference standards for the age group in Europe.

The exercises included a cardiorespiratory fitness test, a 'flamingo' balance test, a handgrip strength test, a standing long jump, a 40m sprint and a sit-and-reach test for flexibility.

The results, published in the *International Journal of Obesity*, found that girls had better balance and flexibility than boys, whilst boys performed better in speed and agility, muscular strength and cardiorespiratory fitness (CRF). Overall, older children performed better than younger children, except for CRF in boys and flexibility in girls.

Low fitness levels during childhood and adolescence are associated with increased future risk of obesity, cardiovascular diseases, impaired skeletal health, reduced quality of life and poor mental health. In spite of the much publicised benefits of being physically active, young people's performance in fitness tests has declined over the last three decades.

Dr Luis Gracia-Marco of the Children's Health and Exercise Research Centre within Sport & Health Sciences at the University of Exeter, one of the study's authors, said: "There is a real scarcity of data on standards of fitness for children. Our study is the first to provide standard values of sex and age-specific fitness for this age group of children in Europe. These values may be useful in identifying those children at higher risk of developing unfavourable health outcomes owing to their low fitness level."

The researchers suggest the data could be useful for schools, sports clubs and other organisations to help classify when a child's performance could indicate that there is a risk to their health in the future. For example, low scores on CRF and handgrip tests are associated with cardiovascular issues.

A total of 10,302 children from eight European countries took part in the study.

11 November 2014

⇨ The above information is reprinted with kind permission from the University of Exeter. Please visit www.exeter.ac.uk for further information.

© University of Exeter 2017

Physical activity levels in children

England	five to 15 (all children)	two to four	five to seven	eight to ten	11–12	13–15
	%	%	%	%	%	%
Boys						
Meeting recommendations	21	9	24	26	19	14
Some activity	41	6	39	40	38	44
Low activity	39	85	37	34	43	42
Base	*643*	*212*	*192*	*175*	*123*	*153*
Girls						
Meeting recommendations	16	10	23	16	14	8
Some activity	40	7	37	41	44	38
Low activity	45	83	40	43	42	54
Base	*651*	*206*	*182*	*190*	*133*	*146*

Source: Physical activity statistics 2015, *British Heart Foundation, February 2015*

Out-of-school activities improve children's educational attainment

Participating in organised sports and joining after-school clubs can help to improve primary school children's academic performance and social skills, new research shows.

Funded by the Nuffield Foundation, researchers from NatCen Social Research, Newcastle University and ASK Research analysed information on more than 6,400 English children born in 2000–01 who are being followed by the Millennium Cohort Study.

Children taking part in organised sports and physical activities at the ages of five, seven and 11 were almost one and a half times more likely to reach a higher than expected level in their Key Stage 2 (KS2) maths test at age 11. No relationship was found between organised sports and activities and KS2 English and science scores.

Among disadvantaged children, those who attended after-school clubs also fared better than their peers who did not take part in such groups. They achieved on average, a two-point higher total score in their KS2 assessments in English, maths and science at the end of primary school.

This is equivalent to two-fifths of the 'attainment gap' between poorer children who score, on average, a total of 53 points at KS2 and those from more affluent homes, who gain 58 points.

The study's lead investigator, Dr Emily Tanner, of NatCen, said: "Results showed that sports clubs were positively associated with attainment outcomes at age 11, even when accounting for prior attainment at age seven.

"For children from economically disadvantaged backgrounds, who have lower take-up of formal out-of-school activities, school-based clubs appear to offer an affordable and inclusive means of supporting academic attainment."

From the ages of five to 11, formal sports club activity was dominated by children from more well-off families. This peaked at age seven with almost four out of five taking part, compared to only two out of five of those from poorer homes.

In comparison, roughly equal numbers of children from both backgrounds were involved in after-school clubs at ages five, seven and eleven.

The researchers also discovered that children who participated in organised sports and physical activities at any time during primary school had better social, emotional and behavioural skills than those who did not take part.

This was also the case for disadvantaged children who had attended an after-school club during primary school, compared with other poorer children who had never joined one.

The findings took into account background factors such as child gender, ethnicity, age and family structure, as well as parental income and occupational class.

Dr Tanner said: "The recent Budget announcement to direct money raised by the tax on sugary drinks towards funding sport and after-school activities suggests policymakers are recognising the wide-ranging benefits of these activities.

"After school clubs, based on school premises, seem to be an easy vehicle for policymakers and educators to ensure that children have access to both the core curriculum and wider enriching activities."

Notes

1. *The study's authors have defined disadvantaged children as those whose family income was below the poverty line (below 60% of the median equivalised household income) in at least two of the three MCS interviews during primary school.*

2. *During the MCS surveys, parents were asked if their child took part in a range of activities outside school lesson time. These included a wide range of organised sports and physical activities, from swimming lessons, dance classes to football training.*

3. *Participating in organised sports and activities had a greater effect than after-school clubs on the assessment scores of more well-off children. After-school group attendance had a greater influence on the test scores of disadvantaged children than those of their more affluent peers.*

4. *The UK national curriculum is organised into blocks of years called 'key stages'. There is a formal assessment at the end of each key stage, which measures children's educational progress compared with other pupils of the same age across the country. Key Stage 2 is the four years of schooling in England and Wales, when pupils are aged between seven and 11. At Key Stage 2 the national expected attainment is level 4.*

5. *The Millennium Cohort Study is following 19,000 young people born across the UK in 2000–01, building a uniquely detailed portrait of the children of the new century. The study is funded by the Economic and Social Research Council and a consortium of government departments, and managed by the Centre for Longitudinal Studies at the UCL Institute of Education. Visit www.cls.ioe.ac.uk/mcs.*

19 April 2016

⇨ The above information is reprinted with kind permission from NatCen Social Research. Please visit www.natcen.ac.uk for further information.

Poor fitness is a bigger threat to child health than obesity

An article from **The Conversation.**

By Gavin Sandercock, Reader in Sports Science (Clinical Physiology), University of Essex

The least fit ten-year-old English child from a class of 30 in 1998 would be one of the five fittest children in the same class tested today. These are the worrying findings of a new piece of research that has crystallised the need to focus on a sharp decline in fitness levels, not obesity, when it comes to improving children's health.

Back in 2009, we reported an 8% decline in fitness of ten-year-old children from the borough of Chelmsford, Essex. At the time this was twice the global rate of fitness decline. The story got a lot of media attention and then chief medical officer Liam Donaldson proposed the introduction of fitness assessments to monitor children's health. But unfortunately he resigned his post soon after and following a change in government, nothing happened and all went quiet. Until now.

This year, the trade body UK Active published its *Generation Inactive* report which contains five recommendations to improve children's health through physical activity. One of these is a repeated call to use fitness measurements to follow trends in physical activity, evaluate trials and tell us more about our children's health.

The next day our follow-up to the 2009 study was published. By testing another 300 ten-year-olds six years later, we confirmed two things. First, there simply is no obesity epidemic – at least not in the schools we visited. Less than 5% of pupils were obese and the average body mass index (BMI) was below 1998 values. This might have been a good news story if BMI was all we had measured; but our fitness test results told a different story.

Thinner, but less puff

A drop in BMI tells us only that the children are "thinner" but tells us nothing about what caused this change. BMI could be lower due to decreased energy intake (food), due to increases in energy expenditure (exercise), or both. One thing we do know is that children with a lower BMI usually do better on the 20m shuttle run used to test their fitness in this experiment because being lighter makes it easier to run and turn. Based on their BMI, we predicted that our 2014 sample would out-perform the relatively heavier children we had measured six years ago.

Yet despite a lower BMI, the 2014 children still couldn't run as fast as their classmates from 2008. The overall rate of decline was 0.95% per year; faster than the 0.8% per year decline from 1998–2008.

Fitness has been declining even faster over the past six years than in the decade before. Girl's fitness fell at twice the global average but our data showed boys' fitness is declining three times faster in England than it is in the rest of the world.

Analysing pupils' actual test performance (how many shuttles they run) shows just how big the fall in fitness from 1998 to 2014 is. In 1998, the average boy ran 60 shuttles (1.2km) before stopping; in 2014, they ran only 33 (660 m). To put this in context, in 1998 the average boy could run a mile in seven minutes 50 seconds but it would take boys today nine minutes and 40 seconds. That's nearly two minutes slower. Girls are also one minute 40 seconds slower than in 1998, and it would now take the average girl over ten minutes to cover a mile.

Our fitness data also told us why the BMI had gone down. By process of elimination, it could not be that children were expending more energy by being more active as this would have improved, or at least maintained their cardiovascular fitness. Instead, combining our BMI and fitness findings told us that children are eating less and doing less exercise.

Low activity levels won't come as a surprise: national surveys repeatedly show an inactivity pandemic; however, the idea that children are eating less might. We purchase around 30% fewer calories today than 20 years ago and there is evidence we've been eating less and less since the 1970s. Given the current hysteria over sugar it's worth mentioning that as well as eating less, the percentage of calories children get from sugar has also declined since the 1990s

BMI isn't everything

English childhood obesity figures reported in the press mostly originate from the National Child Measurement Programme (NCMP). The way these figures are reported artificially inflates the obesity problem for two reasons. First, the NCMP itself uses a rather out-dated definition of obesity (which is not even allowed in some scientific journals). Second, headline figures usually combine 'overweight' and 'obese' BMI categories. Overweight is not a health problem, there is growing evidence that adults with a BMI classed as overweight are the most healthy.

Our study has shown that this continued reliance on BMI as the lone measurement of child health is not working. Yet again, we find ourselves calling for a rethink on how we monitor children's health.

We agree with UK Active that there is an acute need to increase the physical activity levels of young people. Yet activity itself is notoriously difficult to measure. Fitness is the single most important indicator of someone's health and can be measured safely and objectively in the general population. Perhaps most importantly, and unlike weight or BMI, fitness is very sensitive to changes in physical activity behaviour. You may know (or be) someone who has found it hard to lose weight, but have you ever met anyone who didn't get any fitter when they started exercising?

The UK spent just nearly £9 billion on hosting the 2012 Olympics hoping to "inspire a generation" but we have no idea if this has had any effect on children's health or fitness. The Government is currently investing £150 million annually through the primary school PE and sport premium but again, no one is evaluating whether this is going to have any impact on children's health and fitness.

Six years since it was first proposed, the need to systematically assess children's health-related fitness seems greater than ever. The need to drastically increase children's physical activity levels is even more pressing but it is only through measurement and evaluation that we can see what works. UK Active has put it better than I ever could:

Measurement is the first step that leads to control and eventually to improvement. If you can't measure something, you can't understand it. If you can't understand it, *you can't control it. If you can't control it, you can't improve it.*

22 June 2015

⇨ The above information is reprinted with kind permission from *The Conversation*. Please visit www.theconversation.com for further information.

"Fat but fit" counts for nothing scientists say – obesity is what drives early death

Obese people who regularly exercise are far more likely to die early, compared with slim people who take little or no exercise, research suggests.

By Laura Donnelly, Health Editor

Scientists say they have bust the myth that you can be "fat but fit" with research showing obese regular exercisers are likely to die before slim unfit people.

The study of 1.3 million men found that obese people with high levels of aerobic fitness were 30 per cent more likely to die prematurely, compared with those were slim, despite taking little exercise.

The Swedish research tracked men for 30 years, before coming to the conclusion that being the right weight is the most important factor for long-term health.

Scientists said the findings, published in the *International Journal of Epidemiology*, demolished the myth that being fit was sufficient to protect health, and could compensate for obesity.

A number of studies have suggested that obese people who were regular exercisers were at no greater risk of a potentially fatal illness than normal weight people.

The new research, the largest study of its kind, was based on 18-year-old Swedish military conscripts whose aerobic fitness was tested by asking them to cycle until they had to stop due to fatigue.

They were then followed into middle age, for an average of 29 years.

Prof. Peter Nordstrom, of Umea University, Sweden, said: "Unfit normal-weight individuals had 30 per cent lower risk of death from any cause than did fit obese individuals."

He said the findings challenged the idea that obese people could compensate for their mortality risk by taking plenty of exercise.

Prof. Nordstrom added: "These results suggest low BMI (body mass index) early in life is more important than high physical fitness, with regard to reducing the risk of early death."

Overall, men in the highest fifth of aerobic fitness had a 48 per cent lower risk of death from any cause compared with those in the lowest fifth.

Such men had an 80 per cent lower chance of death associated with alcohol or drug abuse, a 59 per cent lower chance of suicide, with a 45 per cent drop in heart disease deaths.

But when such men were obese, being a regular exerciser carried no advantage – such cases were still much more likely to die early compared with slim men.

Around two thirds of Britons are overweight or obese.

Earlier this month England's chief medical officer suggested obesity poses such a threat to the country that it should be treated as a "national risk" alongside terrorism.

Prof. Dame Sally Davies urged women in particular to take steps to slim down – warning that rising levels of obesity in pregnancy are jeopardising the health of future generations.

She said that the problem is becoming so deadly that it is now threatening to overwhelm the NHS and cripple society's productivity.

Next month the Government will publish its childhood obesity strategy, which is expected to pledge restrictions on marketing and advertising of unhealthy foods to children.

However, David Cameron has so far resisted calls for the introduction of a 'sugar tax' on sugary drinks and foods.

Tam Fry, from the National Obesity Forum, said: "Fatness and inactivity are separate but related risk factors, which both increase mortality. So to have one or the other is always bad but to have both is critical."

21 December 2015

⇨ The above information is reprinted with kind permission from *The Telegraph*. Please visit www.telegraph.co.uk for further information.

Poorer people are less physically active

Rising inactivity and obesity increases the risk of chronic ill health, with subsequent large costs to individuals and society. However, physical inactivity is not just a public health problem, but is also connected to economic and cultural issues. Gaining a better understanding of who is physically inactive is essential to designing effective policy interventions to reverse the numbers.

Researchers from the ESRC Centre for Market and Public Organisation (CMPO) and colleagues from Monash, RMIT Melbourne and Lancaster universities examined data on over one million adults in England using the Active People Surveys. The large sample size and detailed local information made it possible to produce precise estimates of the link between physical inactivity and different aspects of individual socio-economic positions, adjusted for local cost of physical activity.

Their research shows high levels of inactivity are closely associated with people's socio-economic position – specifically income, education and local area deprivation. Other factors influencing physical activity include gender, ethnic group, age and geographic area.

Physical activity has a direct cost in terms of money and time which is higher for the poor than the well-off. The costs of physical activity will also be determined in part by where individuals work and live; low-income areas may have smaller tax funds to provide recreation and other facilities for exercise, and higher crime rates can also make physical activity more difficult.

The findings indicate that England is developing a large future health problem which is heavily graded along a socio-economic scale. The large socio-economic gaps suggest that the many current campaigns may not be reaching those who need them most. Unless behaviour patterns are altered, the health disparities are likely to grow.

Key findings

Levels of physical inactivity in England are very high; nearly 80 per cent of the population do not hit key national government targets.

Education, household income and local area deprivation are all independently associated with inactivity. These differences are already evident in young adults, and increase steadily with age.

Females, ethnic minorities, and people in low socio-economic positions are all less likely to do any activity than males, people classifying themselves as White, and those with the highest socio-economic positions.

Inactivity increases the more people are disadvantaged in socio-economic terms. Even low-cost activities such as walking are affected by socio-economic position, and the difference increases with increasing activity cost.

Local area facilities and geographical factors explain very little of the variation in physical inactivity in England; the variations are primarily associated with individual and household characteristics.

Policy relevance and implications

Including more physical activity in the school curriculum and improving school facilities may help cross socio-economic divides early in life.

More targeted health education in certain key groups may help, in order to raise awareness of inactivity as the most important risk factor which can be modified for chronic illness.

Subsidising sports centres and swimming pools to keep prices low could enable low-income people to attend local facilities.

Financial support for the development of sports facilities in lower socio-economic areas with reduced tax bases could provide gyms, football pitches and pools which are free at the point of access.

February 2014

⇨ The above information is reprinted with kind permission from Economic and Social Research Council. Please visit www.esrc.ac.uk for further information.

© ESRC 2017

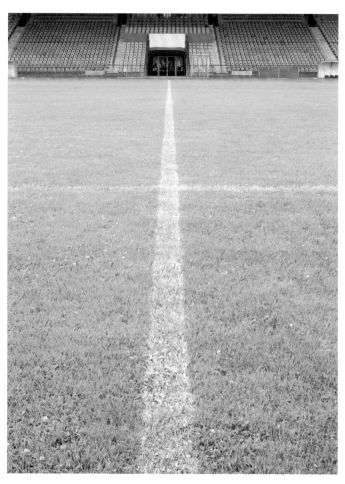

Nearly one in five believe local park threatened

Nearly one in five people (16 per cent) say that their local park or green space is currently or has previously been under threat of being lost or built on, according to a new survey by Fields in Trust.[1]

Nearly all (95%) agree that parks and play areas should be protected from development and 82 per cent feel so strongly that they would be motivated to campaign against a park loss. Two thirds (69%) state that the loss of parks would be detrimental to children's development and half of respondents admitted that they would be less active if their local green space was lost.

The research found almost half of people say using their local park helps them to feel healthier (48%), with 70% of 16- to 24-year-olds also feeling less stressed as a result of having access to green space. Spending quality time with the family and feeling part of a community were also identified as important. Nearly a quarter of people (24%) use their local park at least twice a week.

Fields in Trust currently safeguards over 2,500 sites; a total of 28,000 acres of land including playgrounds, playing fields, and formal and informal parkland across the UK.

As part of its work, Fields in Trust has supported practitioners since the 1930s on open space provision and design. On Thursday 5 November, the charity will launch its latest provision guide, *Guidance for Outdoor Sport and Play: Beyond the Six Acre Standard,* at the House of Lords. The guide will act as a crucial tool for local planning authorities, developers, planners, urban designers and landscape architects in the planning and design of outdoor sport, play and informal open space.

Helen Griffiths, Fields in Trust Chief Executive, said: "These findings demonstrate to us that people really value their local green spaces, with three quarters telling us that they Nearly all agree that parks and play areas should be protected from development and would feel unhappy if their local park was built on or closed tomorrow. We live in a fast-paced world and access to green space provides us all with a chance to take time-out and spend quality time being active with friends and family.

"Whilst we already protect a huge number of spaces across the country, more can be done. People often assume that their local park will always be there but this isn't necessarily the case. The first step in getting a park protected is often for local people to actively campaign for it. Today we are encouraging people to take the first step by visiting our website to find out if their favourite local park is safe."

Fields in Trust ambassador and former England footballer, Graeme Le Saux, said: "I was born and grew up in Jersey, where I had unlimited access to outdoor space, whether it was playing fields, parks or sand dunes. Without this, I would never have had the opportunity to have a career in football. It's these places that cemented my interest in sport and ultimately enabled me to develop my skills."

The most regular park users are those in the North East, with one in five visiting their local open space almost daily. This is closely followed by Londoners, where almost a third of people use their park between one to three times a week. Going for walks (62%), relaxing (31%) and walking the dog (24%), were accounted as the main reasons for people visiting their local park.

Fields in Trust's annual awards ceremony in December celebrates the great work being done in parks and playgrounds across the UK. This year, for the first time, the Fields in Trust Awards will feature a special category 'UK's Best Park' that will be entirely voted for by the public. Voting is now open and everyone is invited to nominate their favourite local green space, whether that's a park, sports field, playground or something else entirely.

Fields in Trust Chief Executive Helen Griffiths said: "Our research shows that the nation's parks and green spaces are places to enjoy life experiences, with many of those surveyed saying that's where they taught their grandchildren to cycle, had their first kiss or reached a personal sporting milestone. Some people have even experienced or witnessed a marriage proposal!

"Our awards help recognise the role that our parks play in our communities, bringing people together and creating a safe outdoor environment that everyone should be entitled to. As Fields in Trust celebrates its 90th year we invite all park users to vote for their favourite green space."

Research methodology

Censuswide interviewed a random sample of 2,079 UK adults between 13 October 2015 and 20 October 2015.

About Fields in Trust

Fields in Trust is a national charity that operates throughout the UK to safeguard recreational spaces and campaign for better statutory protection for all kinds of outdoor sites.

⇨ The above information is reprinted with kind permission from Fields in Trust. Please visit www.fieldsintrust.org for further information.

© Fields in Trust 2017

1   Censuswide, 2,079 UK adults, 13 October 2015 to 20 October 2015.

Fitness sector primed for substantial growth: ukactive report

Consumer thirst for fitness will see gym sector become 'shining star' of post-Brexit economy.

The value of the UK gym sector is set to increase by £1.1 billion in 2016, driven by a hive of investment activity amid growing consumer appetite for fitness, according to a new financial report from non-profit health body ukactive.

Released today (18 October), *The Rise of the Activity Sector* report spotlights the UK's fast-changing fitness landscape and predicts it to grow by 17 per cent in 2016. Valuation specialist Mazars and sponsorship experts Nielsen Sports conducted analyses for the report, which estimates the gym sector will be worth £7.7 billion by the end of 2016 (up from £6.6 billion last year) as investors are enticed by the sector's strong growth prospects.

Low-cost giant The Gym Group floated on the London Stock Exchange last year, while the UK's largest fitness chain Pure Gym has recently sought to follow suit, with several other operators expected to go public in the mid-term as they seek financial backing to fuel rapid expansion.

Despite Pure Gym opting to pull back last week from its planned flotation due to current volatility in the IPO market, the ukactive report underlines the latent potential in the fitness market and points to strong consumer demand as evidence that the sector won't be thrown off course by the choppy waters of Brexit.

Britain's growing gym market is already the largest in Europe and the report tips the sector to be among the 'shining stars' of the UK's post-Brexit economy. British firms accounted for six of the 19 mergers and acquisitions to take place in the European fitness market last year and the UK's position as a hub of investment activity has continued with the recent acquisition of Fitness First UK by Dave Whelan's DW Fitness.

Market segmentation

With 14.3 per cent of UK adults now owning gym memberships – a figure which has increased every year since 2008 – the report sheds light on the growing appeal of exercise. New concepts have opened the market to a broader range of consumers and there are now 6,435 gyms across the private, public and third sectors, serving 9.2 million members. Official figures show that going to the gym has been a consistent driver of activity participation, with the most recent Sport England statistics showing a seven per cent increase over the last year.

The report charts the rise of the low-cost sector, led by Pure Gym and The Gym Group, who have been credited with 'democratising fitness'. Offering lower prices, 24-hour access and shorter-term contracts, low-cost gyms have played a key role in removing many of the traditional barriers to owning memberships.

At the other end of the spectrum, premium operators such as David Lloyd Leisure, Nuffield Health and Virgin Active have refined their propositions by investing in family friendly full-service offerings. The ukactive report also examines the growing prominence of boutique fitness studios such as Heartcore and Barry's Bootcamp, which offer high-end fitness experiences on a pay-as-you-play basis.

Growth opportunities

In an ageing society where the NHS is being stretched to its limits by preventable lifestyle-related conditions such as heart disease and type 2 diabetes, the report explores how the sector's growth prospects will be further enhanced by the need for practical health policies focused on prevention over cure. Physical inactivity currently costs the UK £20 billion and the Government has started to place greater emphasis on the importance of getting Britons moving more through its recent Sport and Childhood Obesity strategies.

Another focus for the new Government is driving productivity and the report tips the growth of workplace health and well being programmes – key to reducing absenteeism and boosting bottom line – as a major opportunity for the gym sector moving forward.

Technology drivers

The ukactive report notes how one of the big drivers of gym sector growth in recent

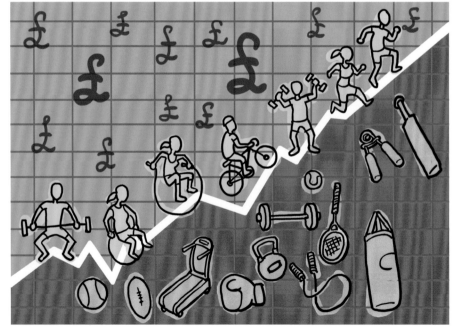

years has been the boom in fitness-focused technology, with giants such as Apple, Microsoft and Google helping to fuel the rise of the "Quantified Self". New products, such as fitness apps and wearable technology, have enhanced the consumer fitness experience, fostering greater engagement and helping to increase gym retention rates.

Landmark report

Accounting for stronger investment sentiment as well as the sponsorship value of gyms, the ukactive report offers a significantly higher valuation of the sector than previous reports. It notes that economic value and growth is being driven by more than rising revenues, with market segmentation, technology and increasingly diverse consumers (such as older females and over 65s) also making an impact.

In addition to its valuation forecast, *The Rise of the Activity Sector* report highlights 15 case studies from organisations which have shaped the 'coming of age' of the sector.

Nick Bishop, Managing Director, Morgan Stanley, Head of Leisure EMEA, said: "As we can see from the flurry of recent investment activity, there is significant investor interest in the physical activity sector, driven by strong growth prospects.

"For now the focus in the UK has been mainly on the low-cost segment, the growth of which has been driven by existing fitness members seeking value and new fitness members attracted by the low entry price.

"Exercise has a major role to play in the health agenda and the sustained increases in gym memberships since 2008 and the sector's relative resilience following that turbulent period shows that it is becoming increasingly ingrained as a positive habit in the lives of UK consumers."

Steven Ward, Executive Director of ukactive, said: "Britain is waking up to the benefits of physical activity and eagle-eyed investors have been quick to spot the sector's potential.

"This report is the first to highlight the true economic value of the health and fitness sector and show that the UK's gyms are very much open for business.

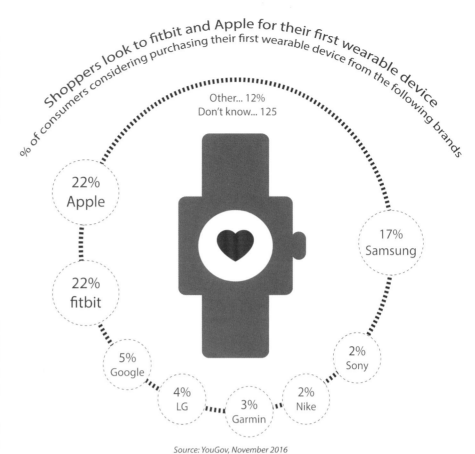

Source: YouGov, November 2016

"Having boosted memberships throughout the recession, we expect gyms to be among the shining stars of Britain's post-Brexit economy, driving substantial business growth while keeping the national healthy, happy and productive."

John Treharne, CEO of The Gym Group, said:

"The Gym Group was conceived in the teeth of the last recession and has since grown to 82 gyms with over 420,000 members. We've played a leading role in the rise of the low-cost sector and 30 per cent of our new members have never joined a gym before, which has been key to broadening the market.

"As ever, location, quality of gym equipment, convenient opening hours, ease of joining, highly flexible contract and good changing facilities are all key to success in this fast-growing market.

"Research suggests there remains significant capacity for more gyms in the UK and we are confident that the low-cost sector will remain a major driver of growth with the market yet to reach maturity."

Matt Merrick, investor and adviser to the health and wellbeing sector and former Virgin Active COO, said:

"The health, fitness and activity landscape is likely to attract significant investment interest over the coming years. Favourable demographic and sociological trends make investing in this space particularly appealing in the medium to long term as people increasingly focus on their health, fitness and longevity.

"The health and fitness market is on the brink of a digital and customer experience revolution and this disruption will not only offer M&A opportunities within the existing operator landscape, it will also see the rise of an emerging start-up community who create unique and engaging experiences which grow the market overall."

"Investors need to have a clear plan as to how they intend to realise a return for their shareholders. The hunters will inevitably become the hunted if they fail to keep ahead of the curve on technology and customer experience developments."

17 October 2016

⇨ The above information is reprinted with kind permission from ukactive. Please visit www.ukactive.com for further information.

Chapter 2

Understanding obesity

About obesity

The epidemic of obesity is now recognised as one of the most important public health problems facing the world today. Tragically, adult obesity is more common globally than under-nutrition. According to the World Health Organization (2014), there are around two billion adults overweight, of those 670 million are considered to be affected by obesity (BMI ≥30 kg/m^2) and 98 million severely affected by obesity (BMI ≥35 kg/m^2). If current trends continue it is estimated that 2.7 billion adults will be overweight, over one billion affected by obesity and 177 million adults severely affected by obesity by 2025.

We estimate that around 224 million school-age children are overweight, making this generation the first predicted to have a shorter lifespan than their parents.

What is obesity?

Obesity is a medical condition described as excess body weight in the form of fat. When accumulated, this fat can lead to severe health impairments.

What causes obesity?

Obesity is caused by an energy imbalance; when intake of calories exceeds expenditure of calories, the surplus energy is stored as body weight. There are a multitude of 'obesogenic' factors contributing to the increased energy consumption and decreased energy expenditure that are responsible for obesity, including:

⇨ Declining levels of physical labour as populations move from rural to urban settings and abandon walking in favour of driving, labour-saving devices in the home, and the replacement of active sport and play by television and computer games.

⇨ Higher levels of food consumption, or an increase in energy density (particularly fat content) of the food we eat.

⇨ Social, economic, educational and cultural factors are important underlying causes of obesity, although how they inter-relate to promote or protect against the development of obesity is complex and varies considerably by country.

How is obesity measured?

The most widely-used method of measuring and identifying obesity is Body Mass Index (BMI) (BMI = weight in kg/height in m^2).

Overweight, or pre-obesity, is defined as a BMI of 25–29.9 kg/m^2, while a BMI >30 kg/m^2 defines obesity. These BMI thresholds were proposed by WHO expert reports and reflect the increasing health risk of excess weight as BMI increases above an optimal range of 21–23 kg/m^2, the recommended median goal for adult Caucasian populations (WHO/NUT/NCD, 2000).

While BMI is a simple measure that is very useful for populations, it should be considered a rough guide for predicting risk in individuals. The distribution and amount of body fat are also crucial determinants of some obesity-associated health risks. Visceral fat, particularly in the abdominal region, has a stronger association with type 2 diabetes and cardiovascular disease than BMI. Accordingly, measures of central

Classification	BMI Kg/m^2	
The World Health Organization International Classification of adult underweight, overweight and obesity according to BMI		
	Principal cut off points	**Additional cut off points**
Underweight	<18.50	<18.50
Severe thinness	<16.00	<16.00
Moderate thinness	16.00 – 16.99	16.00 – 16.99
Mild thinness	17.00 – 18.49	17.00 – 18.49
Normal range	18.50 – 24.99	18.50 – 22.99 23.00 – 24.99
Overweight	≥25.00	≥25.00
Pre-Obesity	25.00 – 29.99	25.00 – 27.49 27.50 – 29.99
Obesity	≥30.00	≥30.00
Obesity class I	30.00 – 34-99	30.00 – 32.49 32.50 – 34.99
Obesity class II	35.00 – 39.99	35.00 – 37.49 37.50 – 39.99
Obesity class III	≥40.00	≥40.0

Source: WHO website (http://www.who.int/bmi)

obesity such as waist:hip ratio and waist circumference provide more robust indices of overall obesity-related health risk than BMI alone.

Health impact of obesity

Obesity is an important cause of morbidity, disability and premature death (WHO, 2004). Obesity increases the risk for a wide range of chronic diseases; BMI is thought to account for about 60% of the risk of developing type 2 diabetes, over 20% of that for hypertension and coronary-heart disease and between 10 and 30% for various cancers. Other co-morbidities include gall-bladder disease, fatty liver, sleep apnoea and osteoarthritis.

The disability attributable to obesity and its consequences in 2004 was calculated at over 36 million disability-adjusted life years (DALYs), due primarily to ischaemic heart disease and type 2 diabetes (WHO Global Health Risks Report, 2004).

Obesity shortens life expectancy. In 2004, increased BMI alone was estimated to account for 2.8 million deaths, while the combined total with physical inactivity was 6.0 million (WHO Global Health Risks Report, 2004) – surpassing the excess mortality associated with tobacco, and approaching that of high blood pressure, the top risk factor for death.

Relationships between obesity and health risks vary between populations. Asians, for example, are more susceptible and thus BMI risk thresholds are lower than other populations, with an action point for overweight defined at 23 kg/m^2.

Obesity in children

Childhood obesity is already common, especially in westernised countries. In 2004, according to IOTF criteria, it was estimated that ~10% of children worldwide aged five to 17 years were overweight and that two to 3% were obese (Lobstein et al., 2004). Prevalence rates vary considerably between different regions and countries, from <5% in Africa and parts of Asia to >20% in Europe and >30% in the Americas and some countries in the Middle East. Becoming obese earlier in life clearly

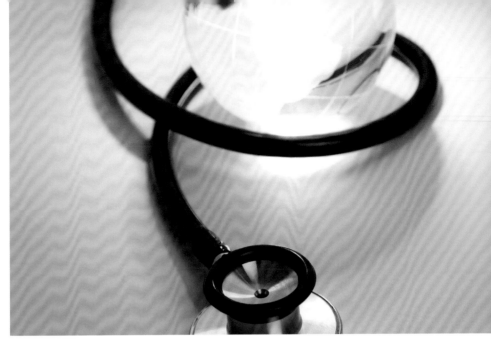

amplifies certain health risks, particularly for type 2 diabetes.

The IOTF criteria for overweight and obesity in children have recently been updated.

Social impact of obesity

For individuals, psychological problems associated with obesity are common, wide-ranging and potentially serious. Growing worldwide awareness of obesity may have reinforced prejudice against the obese, who are often stigmatised. Depression and low self-esteem can affect an individual's quality of life, mental health, educational achievement and employment prospects. Cultural and ethnic factors undoubtedly modulate the social impact of obesity, as well as its perception. In some parts of the world – notably the Pacific Islands and parts of Africa – obesity may still carry historic and cultural connotations of power, beauty and affluence.

Costs of obesity

Obesity has substantial direct and indirect costs that put a strain on healthcare and social resources.

Direct medical costs include preventative, diagnostic and treatment services related to overweight and associated co-morbidities. European nations spend two to 8% of their healthcare budgets on obesity, equating to 0.6% of gross domestic product (GDP) for some (Müller-Riemenschneider, Reinhold, Berghöfer, and Willich, 2008). In the USA,

estimates based on 2008 data indicated that overweight and obesity account for $147 billion in total medical expenditure (Finkelstein, Trogdon, Cohen and Dietz, 2009). Although indirect costs to society can be substantially higher, they are often neglected. They relate to income lost from decreased productivity, reduced opportunities and restricted activity, illness, absenteeism and premature death. In addition, there are high costs associated with the numerous infrastructure changes that societies must make to cope with obese people (i.e. reinforced beds, operating tables and wheel chairs; enlarged turnstiles and seats in sports-grounds and modifications to transport safety standards).

Conclusion

Obesity is now reaching pandemic proportions across much of the world and its consequences are set to impose unprecedented health, financial and social burdens on global society unless effective actions are taken to reverse the trend.

10 October 2015

⇨ The above information is reprinted with kind permission from World Obesity Federation. Please visit www.worldobesity.org for further information.

Causes of obesity

Obesity is generally caused by eating too much and moving too little.

If you consume high amounts of energy, particularly fat and sugars, but don't burn off the energy through exercise and physical activity, much of the surplus energy will be stored by the body as fat.

Calories

The energy value of food is measured in units called calories. The average physically active man needs about 2,500 calories a day to maintain a healthy weight, and the average physically active woman needs about 2,000 calories a day.

This amount of calories may sound high, but it can be easy to reach if you eat certain types of food. For example, eating a large takeaway hamburger, fries and a milkshake can total 1,500 calories – and that's just one meal.

Another problem is that many people aren't physically active, so lots of the calories they consume end up being stored in their body as fat.

Poor diet

Obesity doesn't happen overnight. It develops gradually over time, as a result of poor diet and lifestyle choices, such as:

⇨ **eating large amounts of processed or fast food** – that's high in fat and sugar

⇨ **drinking too much alcohol** – alcohol contains a lot of calories, and people who drink heavily are often overweight

⇨ **eating out a lot** – you may be tempted to also have a starter or dessert in a restaurant, and the food can be higher in fat and sugar

⇨ **eating larger portions than you need** – you may be encouraged to eat too much if your friends or relatives are also eating large portions

⇨ **drinking too many sugary drinks** – including soft drinks and fruit juice

⇨ **comfort eating** – if you have low self-esteem or feel depressed, you may eat to make yourself feel better.

Unhealthy eating habits tend to run in families. You may learn bad eating habits from your parents when you're young and continue them into adulthood.

Lack of physical activity

Lack of physical activity is another important factor related to obesity. Many people have jobs that involve sitting at a desk for most of the day. They also rely on their cars, rather than walking or cycling.

For relaxation, many people tend to watch TV, browse the Internet or play computer games and rarely take regular exercise.

If you're not active enough, you don't use the energy provided by the food you eat, and the extra energy you consume is stored by the body as fat.

The Department of Health recommends that adults do at least 150 minutes (two-and-a-half hours) of moderate-intensity aerobic activity, such as cycling or fast walking, every week. This doesn't need to be done all in one go, but can be broken down into smaller periods. For example, you could exercise for 30 minutes a day for five days a week.

If you're obese and trying to lose weight, you may need to do more exercise than this. It may help to start off slowly and gradually increase the amount of exercise you do each week.

Genetics

Some people claim there's no point trying to lose weight because "it runs in my family" or "it's in my genes".

While there are some rare genetic conditions that can cause obesity, such as Prader-Willi syndrome, there's no reason why most people can't lose weight.

It may be true that certain genetic traits inherited from your parents – such as having a large appetite – may make losing weight more difficult, but it certainly doesn't make it impossible.

In many cases, obesity is more to do with environmental factors, such as poor eating habits learned during childhood.

Medical reasons

In some cases, underlying medical conditions may contribute to weight gain. These include:

⇨ **an underactive thyroid gland (hypothyroidism)** – where your thyroid gland doesn't produce enough hormones

⇨ **Cushing's syndrome** – a rare disorder that causes the over-production of steroid hormones.

However, if conditions such as these are properly diagnosed and treated, they should pose less of a barrier to weight loss.

Certain medicines, including some corticosteroids, medications for epilepsy and diabetes, and some medications used to treat mental illness – including antidepressants and medicines for schizophrenia – can contribute to weight gain.

Weight gain can sometimes be a side effect of stopping smoking.

15 June 2016

⇨ The above information is reprinted with kind permission from NHS Choices. Please visit www.nhs.uk for further information.

Obesity statistics

By Carl Baker and Alex Bate

Obesity among adults, England

According to data from the 2014 Health Survey for England, 24% of adults in England are obese and a further 36% are overweight, making a total of 60% who are either overweight or obese.[1] Of obese adults, seven in ten are Class I obese, with a BMI between 30 and 35. Around one in ten obese adults are morbidly obese, with a BMI above 40.

Trends over the last decade

Between 2005[2] and 2014, the proportion of adults who were either overweight or obese decreased slightly from 60.9% to 60.5%. However, this is due to a fall in the proportion of overweight adults, as the proportion of obese (I–III) adults has risen from 23.4% to 24.8%. The proportion classed as normal has also risen, from 36.9% to 37.9%. Obesity has risen more among women than among men over this period. While the rise since 2005 has been slight, the previous decade saw a greater change – in 1994 around 13% of adults were obese.

Obesity by age

The age group most likely to be overweight or obese is age 75–84, but only by a small margin. Prevalence of overweight and obesity is between 74% and 76% among all age groups from 55 to 84. Age 75–84 is the only category with less than a quarter of adults at normal weight. The adult age group least likely to be obese is 16–24-year-olds, with almost 61% at normal weight and only 32% overweight or obese.

---

1   Health Survey for England, 2014 www.hscic. gov.uk/catalogue/PUB19295

2   The different obesity categories were not measured in 2004

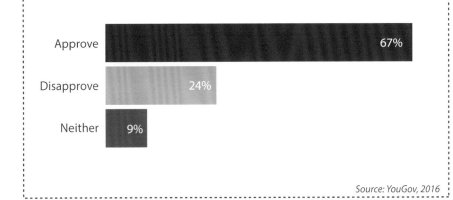

Obese patients wil be refused surgery for up to a year as part of efforts to save money, an NHS commissioing group in North Yorkshire has said. If, however, the patient can shed 10% of their weight, they could be referred within the year. (The new rules will only apply to elective surgery for non-life threatening conditions.)

Do you approve or disapprove?

Approve — 67%
Disapprove — 24%
Neither — 9%

Source: YouGov, 2016

Obesity by gender

Men in England are more likely to be overweight or obese than women. 65% of men were overweight or obese in 2014 compared with 58% of women. Of these, however, 24% of men were obese compared with 27% of women. These proportions vary by age. Only among ages 16–24 are women more likely to be overweight or obese than men. The biggest gap is among 85+-year-olds, with 84% of men overweight and obese compared with 55% of women.

Women are more likely to be morbidly obese than men, across all age groups. 3.6% of women were morbidly obese in 2014, compared to 1.8% of men.

Economic costs of obesity

Estimates of the economic cost of obesity vary and are inherently uncertain. An influential Foresight Report from 2007 estimated that NHS costs attributed to elevated BMI (overweight and obesity) were £4.2 billion in 2007. This was forecast to rise to £6.3 billion in 2015, £8.3 billion in 2025 and £9.7 billion in 2050. This only reflects costs to the health service and not wider economic consequences for society. Estimates of future costs rely on the accuracy of obesity prevalence forecasts.

"Children living in deprived areas are substantially more likely to be obese"

Obesity among children, England

According to data from the National Child Measurement Programme (NCMP), 9% of reception age children (age four to five) are obese, with a further 13% overweight. These proportions are higher among Year 6 children (age ten to 11), with 19% being obese and 14% overweight.

Note that these categories are not directly comparable to those used for adults, since measuring BMI and obesity for children is more complex than for adults. In the NCMP, obese is defined as having a BMI in the 95th percentile or higher of the British 1990 growth reference. Overweight is

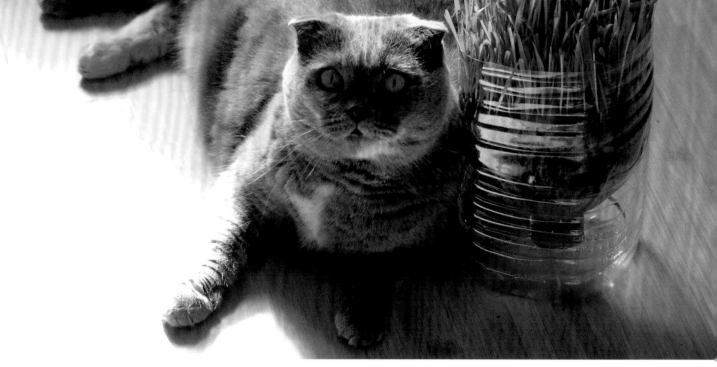

"In England in 2014, pharmacies dispensed just over half a million items for treating obesity with a net ingredient cost of £15.3 million"

defined as a BMI in the 85th percentile or higher.

Small gender differences are present even at age four to five, with 22.6% of boys being overweight or obese compared with 21.2% of girls. At age ten to 11, the gap is wider: 34.9% of boys are overweight or obese compared with 31.5% of girls.

For both reception and Year 6 children, above average obesity is concentrated in parts of London, Birmingham and the Black Country, Merseyside, Manchester, and the North East. Other areas with above average rates for both age groups are: Great Yarmouth, Stoke-on-Trent, Luton, Nottingham and Leicester. Areas with below average obesity rates for both ages tend to be in southern and relatively affluent areas.

Childhood obesity and deprivation

Children living in deprived areas are substantially more likely to be obese. Among reception (age four to five)

children, 5.7% of those in the least deprived areas are obese compared with 12.0% of those in the most deprived areas. In Year 6 (age ten to 11), 11.5% of children in the least deprived areas are obese, compared with 25.0% in the most deprived areas. So in both age groups, children in the most deprived areas are more than twice as likely to be obese. These proportions have changed little since 2010/11.

Children in the most deprived areas are also marginally more likely to be underweight than those in the least deprived areas.

Childhood obesity and ethnicity

According to data from the NCMP, children of Black or Black British ethnicity are most likely to be obese, while children of Chinese or White ethnicity are least likely to be obese. At age four to five (reception), obesity rates among children of Chinese ethnicity are almost half those among children of Black or Black British ethnicity. Between ages four to five and ten to 11, obesity rates among all ethnic groups increase by between nine (White) and 14 (Asian or Asian British) percentage points.

GP prescribing for obesity

In England in 2014, pharmacies dispensed just over half a million

"For both reception and Year 6 children, above average obesity is concentrated in parts of London, Birmingham and the Black Country, Merseyside, Manchester, and the North East"

items for treating obesity with a net ingredient cost of £15.3 million. All of these prescriptions were for Orlistat, which prevents the body from absorbing fat from food. This was a slight fall on the number of prescriptions in 2013, but a rise from 2012 (when there was a stock shortage of Orlistat). Until 2010, Sibumatrine was prescribed in addition to Orlistat, but its marketing authorisation was suspended in the light of concerns that it raised the risk of heart attacks and strokes. Another drug, Rimonabant, was withdrawn in 2009 for related reasons.

2 February 2016

⇨ The above information is reprinted with kind permission from the House of Commons Library. Please visit www.parliament.uk for further information.

Diabetes and obesity

The UK currently ranks as the country with the highest level of obesity in Europe, with more than one in four (28.1%) adults obese and nearly two out of three (63.4%) overweight.

Over the next 20 years, the number of obese adults in the country is forecast to soar to 26 million people.

According to health experts, such a rise would result in more than a million extra cases of type 2 diabetes, heart disease and cancer.

Obesity is also no longer a condition that just affects older people, although the likelihood does increase with age, and increasing numbers of young people have been diagnosed with obesity.

Data from Public Health England suggests that nearly a third (31.2%) of children aged two to 15 years old are obese.

Links between obesity and type 2 diabetes

While the exact causes of diabetes are still not fully understood, it is known that factors up the risk of developing different types of diabetes mellitus.

For type 2 diabetes, this includes being overweight or obese (having a body mass index – BMI – of 30 or greater).

In fact, obesity is believed to account for 80–85% of the risk of developing type 2 diabetes, while recent research suggests that obese people are up to 80 times more likely to develop type 2 diabetes than those with a BMI of less than 22.

How does obesity cause type 2 diabetes?

It is a well-known fact that if you are overweight or obese, you are at greater risk of developing type 2 diabetes, particularly if you have excess weight around your tummy (abdomen).

Inflammatory response

Studies suggest that abdominal fat causes fat cells to release 'pro-inflammatory' chemicals, which can make the body less sensitive to the insulin it produces by disrupting the function of insulin responsive cells and their ability to respond to insulin.

This is known as insulin resistance – the hallmark of type 2 diabetes.

Having excess abdominal fat (i.e. a large waistline) is known as central or abdominal obesity, a particularly high-risk form of obesity.

Disruption in fat metabolism

Obesity is also thought to trigger changes to the body's metabolism. These changes cause fat tissue (adipose tissue) to release fat molecules into the blood, which can affect insulin responsive cells and lead to reduced insulin sensitivity.

Another theory put forward by scientists into how obesity could lead to type 2 diabetes is that obesity causes prediabetes, a metabolic condition that almost always develops into type 2 diabetes.

Preventing obesity

The links between obesity and type 2 diabetes are firmly established – without the intervention of a healthy diet and appropriate exercise, obesity can lead to type 2 diabetes over a relatively short period of time.

The good news is that reducing your body weight, by even a small amount, can help improve your body's insulin sensitivity and lower your risk of developing cardiovascular and metabolic conditions such as type 2 diabetes, heart disease and types of cancer.

According to the NHS, a 5% reduction in body weight followed up by regular moderate intensity exercise could reduce your type 2 diabetes risk by more than 50%.

Cost of obesity

In the UK, the cost to the NHS of obesity and related conditions such as type 2 diabetes is putting a huge, unsustainable drain on NHS resources.

Treating obesity, type 2 diabetes and diabetic complications such as nephropathy, heart disease and amputation is very costly, and with new cases of obesity-related type 2 diabetes soaring each year in the UK, these costs are expected to keep rising.

To tackle this problem, there is a need for widespread and far-reaching culturally appropriate educational literature that informs the population of the risk of eating badly and not taking exercise.

Making lifestyle changes

Making healthy lifestyle changes can often prevent obesity, and in order to avoid a healthcare crisis the UK needs to spread information that highlights the importance of doing just that, especially amongst children.

Obesity facts

⇨ According to the World Health Organization (WHO), at least 2.8 million people are dying each year as a result of being overweight or obese

⇨ In 2008, over 40 million preschool children were overweight worldwide

⇨ The WHO suggests that more than one in four (28.1%) of adults in the UK are obese (has a BMI of 30 or more).

⇨ The UK has the highest level of adult obesity in Europe

⇨ Copeland in Cumbria is the most overweight local authority in England

⇨ Studies into obesity prevention have shown that giving up watching television for a week reduces a child's waist size by an average 2.3cm (just under one inch).

⇨ The above information is reprinted with kind permission from diabetes.co.uk. Please visit www.diabetes.co.uk for further information.

© 2017 Diabetes Digital Media Ltd

Childhood obesity: a plan for action

Introduction

Today nearly a third of children aged two to 15 are overweight or obese[i,1] and younger generations are becoming obese at earlier ages and staying obese for longer.[2] Reducing obesity levels will save lives as obesity doubles the risk of dying prematurely.[3] Obese adults are seven times more likely to become a type 2 diabetic than adults of a healthy weight[4] which may cause blindness or limb amputation. And not only are obese people more likely to get physical health conditions like heart disease, they are also more likely to be living with conditions like depression.[5, 6]

The economic costs are great, too. We spend more each year on the treatment of obesity and diabetes than we do on the police, fire service and judicial system combined.[7] It was estimated that the NHS in England spent £5.1 billion on overweight and obesity-related ill-health in 2014/15.[8]

The burden is falling hardest on those children from low-income backgrounds. Obesity rates are highest for children from the most deprived areas and this is getting worse.[9] Children aged five and from the poorest income groups are twice as likely to be obese compared to their most well-off counterparts and by age 11 they are three times as likely.[10]

Obesity is a complex problem with many drivers, including our behaviour, environment, genetics and culture. However, at its root, obesity is caused by an energy imbalance: taking in more energy through food than we use through activity. Physical activity is associated with numerous health benefits for children, such as muscle and bone strength, health and fitness, improved quality of sleep and maintenance of a healthy weight.[11] There is also evidence that physical activity and

i A child's BMI is based on 'weight for height' defined as weight in kilograms divided by the height in metres squared (kg/m²). To take into account growth patterns by age and gender, children's BMI is compared with CMI centiles on published growth charts. Children with a BMI above the 98th centile are considered clinically obese. For population monitoring those above the 95th centile are classed as obese.

participating in organised sports and after school clubs is linked to improved academic performance.[12, 13]

Long-term, sustainable change will only be achieved through the active engagement of schools, communities, families and individuals.

We aim to significantly reduce England's rate of childhood obesity within the next ten years. We are confident that our approach will reduce childhood obesity while respecting consumer choice, economic realities and, ultimately, our need to eat. Although we are clear in our goals and firm in the action we will take, the launch of this plan represents the start of a conversation, rather than the final word.

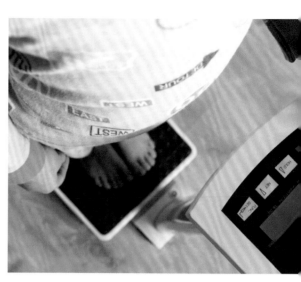

Goals and actions

⇨ Introducing a soft drinks industry levy

⇨ Taking out 20% of sugar in products

⇨ Supporting innovation to help businesses to make their products healthier

⇨ Developing a new framework by updating the nutrient profile model

⇨ Making healthy options available in the public sector

⇨ Continuing to provide support with the cost of healthy food for those who need it most

⇨ Helping all children to enjoy an hour of physical activity every day

⇨ Improving the co-ordination of quality sport and physical activity programmes for schools

⇨ Creating a new healthy rating scheme for primary schools

⇨ Making school food healthier

⇨ Clearer food labelling

⇨ Supporting early years settings

⇨ Harnessing the best new technology

⇨ Enabling health professionals to support families.

Conclusion

With nearly a third of children aged two to 15 overweight or obese[14], tackling childhood obesity requires us all to take action. Government, industry, schools and the public sector all have a part to play in making food and drink healthier and supporting healthier choices for our children. The benefits for reducing obesity are clear – it will save lives and reduce inequalities.

The actions in this plan will significantly reduce England's rate of childhood obesity within the next ten years. Achieving this will mean fewer obese children in 2026 than if obesity rates stay as they are.[15]

References

1 Health and Social Care Information Centre (2015) Health Survey for England 2014.

2 Johnson W, Li L, Kuh D, Hardy R (2015) How Has the Age-Related Process of Overweight or Obesity Development Changed over Time? Coordinated Analyses of Individual Participant Data from Five United Kingdom Birth Cohorts. PLoS Med 12(5).

3 T. Pischon MD et al. (2008) General and Abdominal Adiposity and Risk of Death in Europe. The New England Journal of Medicine. 359:2105-2120.

4 Asnawi Abdullah, Anna Peeters, Maximilian de Courten, Johannes Stoelwinder (2010) The magnitude of association between overweight and obesity and the risk of diabetes: A metaanalysis of prospective cohort studies. Diabetes Research and Clinical Practice.

5 Health and Social Care Information Centre (2015) Health Survey for England 2014.

6 Gatineau M, Dent M (2011) Obesity and Mental Health. Oxford: National Obesity Observatory.

7 McKinsey Global Institute (2014) Overcoming Obesity: An Initial Economic Analysis.

8 Estimates for UK in 2014/15 are based on: Scarborough, P. (2011) The economic burden of ill health due to diet, physical inactivity, smoking, alcohol and obesity in the UK: an update to 2006–07 NHS costs. Journal of Public Health. May 2011, 1-9. Uplifted to take into account inflation. No adjustment has been made for slight changes in overweight and obesity rates over this period. It's been assumed England costs account for around 85% of UK costs.

9 Health and Social Care Information Centre (2015) National Child Measurement Programme, England 2014/15.

10 Yvonne Kelly, Alice Goisis, and Amanda Sacker (2015) Why are poorer children at higher risk of obesity and overweight? A UK cohort study. The European Journal of Public Health.

11 Start Active, Stay Active: A report on physical activity from the four home countries' Chief Medical Officers, July 2011.

12 PHE (2014) The link between pupil health and wellbeing and attainment https://www.gov.uk/government/ uploads/system/uploads/attachment_data/file/370686/HT_briefing_layoutvFINALvii.pdf.

13 Chanfreau et al. (2016) Out of school activities during primary school and KS2 attainment.

14 Health and Social Care Information Centre (2015) Health Survey for England 2014.

15 There are 1.6 million obese children aged 2-15 in England: Health and Social Care Information Centre (2015) Health Survey for England 2014 Trend Tables.

August 2016

⇨ The above information is reprinted with kind permission from the House of Commons Library. Please visit www.parliament.uk for further information.

What does obesity cost the economy?

By Laura O'Brien

In brief

Claim

Obesity costs the economy £27 billion a year.

Conclusion

This is the best estimate we've got of the total cost of obesity and being overweight to the NHS and the economy. But it's based on analysis that's over a decade old and there's a lot of uncertainty to the numbers.

"Obesity drives disease. It increases the risk of cancer, diabetes and heart disease – and it costs our economy £27 billion a year"

George Osborne, 16 March 2016

Announcing a tax on sugary drinks companies yesterday, the Chancellor said it would help to prevent obesity, which he said costs the economy £27 billion a year.

£27 billion may be the best estimate we've got for the total costs to the NHS and the economy of people considered to be overweight and obese in England, but there are issues with it. We don't know enough to be as precise as saying the cost is £27 billion.

Some of the research underpinning the figure is over a decade old. Patterns of obesity may have changed since then, and the economy definitely has. It also relied on some assumptions that were uncertain at the time.

Where the figure comes from

The Government takes its estimate of £27 billion from the National Obesity Observatory, now part of Public Health England.

This took the figure from 2007 research, which in turn based its calculations in part on 2004 research by Parliament's Health Committee.

The 2004 research put the total cost of people considered obese at between £3.3 billion and 3.7 billion in 2002. That was made up of the cost of treating obesity and its consequences – about £1 billion – and the earnings lost due to sickness and premature mortality among obese people.

It said that "if in crude terms" the cost of people considered overweight was half that of people considered obese, and given that there are about twice as many people who are overweight as obese, the total costs of both overweight and obese people would be about £6.6–7.4 billion a year. So about £7 billion.

So the research found the total costs of people being overweight or obese (£7 billion) were seven times the costs of treating obese patients (£1 billion).

The more recent estimate from 2007 is based on the assumption that the total costs of people considered to be overweight or obese continue to be seven times the cost of NHS treatment.

It estimated that the cost of treating obesity alone would be £3.9 billion by 2015, based on projections of the population's body mass index profile, the effect this would have on diseases in the population, and the cost to the NHS of treating these diseases.

It multiplied this £3.9 billion by seven to reach the estimate that the total cost would be £27 billion by 2015.

A lot can change in a decade

Changes in diet since these estimates were made could have affected the number of overweight people, which in turn could have increased or reduced the costs to the NHS and to the economy. The cost of NHS care could have deviated from the forecast for other reasons – for example if drugs costs went up faster than expected.

Similarly, it's not clear that total costs were or will always be seven times the cost to the NHS, as they – roughly – were deemed to be in 2002.

For instance, changes to the labour market and to the benefits system could change the employment rate for people considered to be overweight or obese. That means the overall economic cost could change relative to the treatment costs.

As the National Obesity Observatory said of the research:

"Whilst modelling is helpful, it necessarily relies on existing patterns of treatment and assumptions about continued patterns of eating and physical activity as well as behavioural and social responses to obesity. It might also be helpful to look at alternative scenarios as part of modelling estimates such as: obesity trends continue; obesity continues to rise by a specified percentage per year; obesity is reduced by a specified percentage per year."

Finally, the £27 billion was in 2007 prices. In today's prices the cost would be higher.

17 March 2016

⇨ The above information is reprinted with kind permission from Full Fact. Please visit www.fullfact.org for further information.

URMC study shows obesity diagnosis is often overlooked

Failure to identify obesity results in missed opportunity to intervene.

Despite a growing epidemic, many medical providers fail to diagnose obesity in their patients and miss an opportunity to identify an important component of long-term health, according to a University of Rochester Medical Center study published in the *Journal of Community Health*.

Among patients whose body mass index (BMI) indicated obesity, providers diagnosed and documented obesity in less than a quarter of office visits with children, and less than half for adolescents and adults, researchers found. The study further found that patients living in less-educated communities were even less likely to receive an accurate diagnosis.

"As a medical community, we can't effectively manage obesity until we are identifying it properly in our patients," said Robert J Fortuna, M.D., M.P.H., assistant professor of Medicine and Pediatrics in Primary Care at URMC and one of the study's authors. "By not accurately diagnosing obesity, we are missing the opportunity to influence the trajectory of our patients' health over the course of their lives."

Using data from the National Center for Health Statistics, researchers looked at records from 885,291,770 medical office visits for adults and children from 2006 to 2010. Of the visits where a BMI measurement suggested obesity, the diagnosis of obesity was made in only 23.4 per cent of children ages 5 to 12 years, and 39.7 per cent of adolescents (ages 13 to 21 years). Rates of diagnosis were highest for young adults (ages 22 to 34) at 45.4 per cent, and adults ages 35 to 64 at 43.9 per cent. Adults age 65 and older were diagnosed as obese 39.6 per cent of the time. Obesity was more likely to be identified in females and in people who live in areas with a higher percentage of college-educated adults.

The study echoes previous research that demonstrates that up to 82 per cent of children and young adults are not being appropriately diagnosed as obese during office visits. The researchers speculated on potential explanations for the failure to diagnose obesity, including the possibility that the high prevalence of obesity in lower socioeconomic areas may desensitise providers to normal body size. In addition, other medical problems and social issues may take priority over discussing obesity, and social stigma may make providers hesitant to label patients, especially children, as obese.

"Discussing obesity with patients must be done in a sensitive and delicate manner; providers may avoid it because they don't want to offend patients," said study co-author Bryan Stanistreet, M.D. "Beyond that, providers may also avoid this discussion because communities lack resources to help support patients, educate them on diet and encourage regular exercise."

"The lower recognition of obesity in vulnerable populations is particularly concerning," Fortuna said. "Our findings demonstrate the fundamental need to improve the recognition of obesity in vulnerable populations, such as young children and those living in less-educated communities."

Erica O. Miller, M.D., Emily Ruckdeschel, M.D., and Karen Nead, M.D., were also co-authors on the study. "Factors Associated with the Accurate Diagnosis of Obesity" was published online in June and will appear in an upcoming print edition of the *Journal for Community Health*.

29 August 2016

⇨ The above information is reprinted with kind permission from the University of Rochester. Please visit www.urmc.rochester.edu for further information.

Hawaiian Airlines to keep assigning flyers' seats based on weight distribution

Airline policy, which began earlier this month, faced federal complaints that it was discriminatory toward people of Samoan descent.

By Martin Pengelly

Hawaiian Airlines will continue assigning seats on some flights according to weight distribution, after complaints to federal authorities that the policy is discriminatory to people of Samoan descent were turned down.

The airline instituted the measure earlier this month, after a survey was carried out because actual fuel consumption had been noticed to be greater than projected fuel consumption on flights from Honolulu to Pago Pago, in American Samoa.

The six-month voluntary passenger survey showed that the average traveller and their luggage weighed 30lb (14kg) more than the airline's estimate.

"What they're saying is Samoans are obese," one man told the Associated Press at Honolulu international airport earlier in October.

In response, Hawaiian Airlines' chief operating officer, Jon Snook, said: "That's an entirely incorrect assumption."

Six complaints were filed with the US transportation department. The complaints were denied, a spokesman told the AP last week, leaving American Samoa as the only Hawaiian Airlines flight without seat pre-selection.

Once passengers have checked in for Hawaiian Airlines, flights to Pago Pago they are allocated seats in a pattern designed to manage weight distribution.

In a 'frequently asked questions' post on its website, the airline said: "Using the new weights, a full row of adults may theoretically exceed the load limitations of the floor in a row in extreme circumstances (such as a crash landing). Keeping one seat open or ensuring a seat is filled with a child mitigates that risk."

Hawaiian Airlines told the AP it had conducted weight surveys on other flights, but had not found evidence that excess weight was a problem.

In its FAQ post, the airline said: "We have done similar weight surveys in our Asian markets, where the average weight was lower than assumed. This is also important to know for weight and balance issues."

The airline is not the first to use weight to determine seating: Samoa Air started charging according to weight in 2013.

Then, Samoa Air's chief executive, Chris Langton, told CNN: "The next step is for the industry to make those sort of changes and recognise that, hey, we are not all 72kg (160lb) any more and we don't all fit into a standard seat.

"What makes airplanes work is weight. We are not selling seats, we are selling weight."

According to the CIA world fact book, *American Samoa* has the highest rate of adult obesity in the world, with Samoa sixth. The top nine countries on the list are Pacific islands, with Kuwait 10th.

Samoa, Fiji and Tonga are leading exporters of rugby players, mostly to Australia, New Zealand and Europe.

Tonga, which has a population of a little over 106,500, supplied players to seven other teams at the 2015 World Cup, among them the England forwards Mako and Billy Vunipola and the Wales No 8 Taulupe Faletau. The double World Cup-winning New Zealand flanker Jerome Kaino was born in Faga'alu, in American Samoa.

Stereotypes of people from Pacific island nations as large, obese and

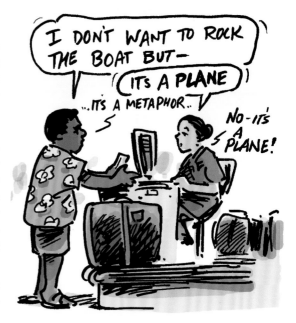

strong have become a world issue not just through rugby, but with the approaching release of *Moana*, an animated Disney movie which features Maui, a Polynesian god.

Jenny Salesa, a New Zealand politician of Tongan heritage, said recently the Maui character had been made to look "half-pig, half-hippo".

Hawaiian Airlines operates one plane, an Airbus A330, that is decorated with the characters from *Moana*.

*This article was amended on 27 October 2016. It initially stated in error that Hawaiian Airlines was "choosing flyers' seats based on their weights". The seating policy for flights to Pago Pago is based on weight distribution. The story also stated in error that passengers would be weighed before flying.

23 October 2016

⇨ The above information is reprinted with kind permission from *The Guardian*. Please visit www.theguardian.com for further information.

© 2017 Guardian News and Media Limited

The importance of overcoming stigma

Important points needing urgent attention.

People who are overweight or living with obesity are often targets of bias and hurtful stigmatisation. This badly affects their daily lives, threatening their health, generating health inequalities, and interfering with effective obesity intervention.

Stigma can lead to avoidance of treatment, increase of eating disorders and decrease of physical activity, depression and even risk of suicide.

There are five important points that need urgent attention:

1. Respect towards patients living with obesity

Patients living with obesity often complain that they are not treated respectfully. People living with obesity should be protected from abuse on all levels. This is true for adults, but also for children and adolescents.

There is an urgent need for greater respect from politicians, healthcare workers, scientists, media, schools and from everyone generally who are inclined to stigmatise people living with obesity.

2. Acceptance that obesity is not a lifestyle choice

Obesity is frequently regarded as a lifestyle choice, even amongst patients themselves, their families and friends. This discourages many patients from seeking medical advice.

It originates from poor knowledge about obesity as a chronic disease. There are many factors that can cause obesity which are beyond someone's control. These include genetic and endocrine conditions, environmental factors such as stress, living in an obesogenic environment and the increasingly sedentary lifestyle patterns that many people now lead.

3. Recognition of obesity as a chronic disease

Obesity needs to be recognised as a chronic disease across all member states of the European Union. Currently only one country, Portugal, recognises obesity as such. This is despite the fact that it is recognised as a disease by the World Health Organization (WHO). Left untreated, obesity causes numerous other diseases including type 2 diabetes, cardiovascular disease and certain types of cancer and depression.

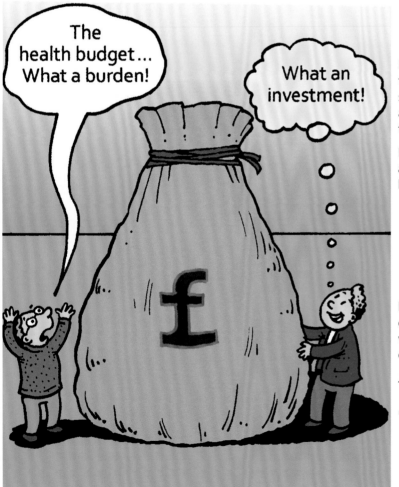

4. Impartial and transparent discussion

Financial concerns are becoming a more important issue than the well-being of patients. This is due to influential stakeholders including industry, media and governments avoiding the discussion of obesity and the stigma attached to it.

Healthcare costs need to be regarded as an investment and not as a burden. After all, it is less expensive to address health problems before they lead to other chronic diseases.

5. Reducing stigmatisation and discrimination can improve recovery rates

It is important to create a supportive healthcare environment to ensure the successful treatment of people with obesity. With the right support, people living with obesity can make real progress.

21 May 2016

⇨ The above information is reprinted with kind permission from European Obesity Day, an initiative of European Association for the Study of Obesity (EASO). Please visit www.europeanobesityday.eu for further information.

Physical literacy – the vaccine against the inactivity crisis

By Dean Horridge

Physical literacy is seen as a "vaccine" against the inactivity crisis. If this is the case, why do we have so many children leaving primary school not physically literate?

Physical literacy refers to movement competency; how well can children run, skip, hop, jump, throw and catch. It also refers to motivation and confidence. The better children are at these skills, the more confident they become and the more motivated they are to keep on participating or even try something new. They will also look for opportunities to be active if we allow them to!

For many years we have been disengaging children by making them play sport before they have learnt the fundamental movement skills. It's time to change and develop children's skills and confidence to be physically active. Engaging children in fun activity to get them moving from a young age will keep them motivated and will embed healthy and active habits for life.

It does not need to be over complicated and it is not hard to achieve, we need to keep it simple. We must commit to

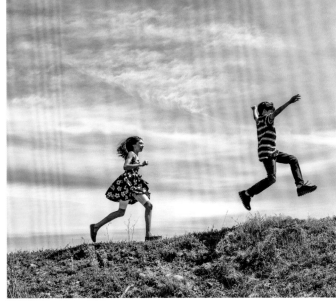

supporting children to achieve the Chief Medical Officer recommended guidelines of 60 minutes activity a day for every child both in and out of school. If we can embed that into schools and communities across the UK, we can tackle the inactivity crisis and obesity epidemic.

Last year, our challenging children's inactivity report highlighted that 67% of children did not have adequate fitness levels for their age. This needs to change and we have an opportunity to make a difference. Let's start today.

For tips and advice to get the whole family moving in ways that can be incorporated into your everyday routine, visit www.activitychallenge.co.uk.

26 April 2016

⇨ The above information is reprinted with kind permission from Fit For Sport. Please visit www.fitforsport.co.uk for further information.

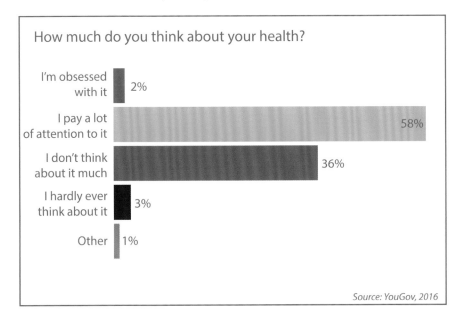

How much do you think about your health?

I'm obsessed with it	2%
I pay a lot of attention to it	58%
I don't think about it much	36%
I hardly ever think about it	3%
Other	1%

Source: YouGov, 2016

How listening to music during exercise can give you a workout boost and make physical activity less painful

From the lyrics to tempo, music can dramatically affect performance by changing a person's mind-set or distracting from discomfort.

By Kashmira Gander

Chances are that the punchy first chords of "Eye of the Tiger", the soundtrack to classic boxing movie *Rocky III*, conjure up images of sporting prowess and success in your mind. It's probably even on your motivational gym playlist to help you pummel the punching bag (don't worry, your secret is safe with us).

Popping ear buds in before a workout is habitual for many of us and exercising without a backing track unthinkable. A recent survey by *Runner's World* found that 75 per cent of respondents consider that jogging to music is beneficial.

Just how music can fuel exercise – when it becomes what is known as an ergogenic aid – is a recent field of scientific study which experts have been exploring for two decades. Their research shows the components of music, from the lyrics to the tempo, can acutely affect performance by changing a person's mind-set or distracting from discomfort, as Dr Costas Karageorghis, reader of sports psychology at Brunel University, argues in his book *Applying Music in Exercise and Sport*.

And it's not just your average runner in the park that relies on the power of music, explains Dr Karageorghis. Even athletes plug in to music to psych themselves up to find that sweet spot known as "the zone".

Studies show that athletes can associate a specific piece of music with the optimum state of mind for exercise over time. In fact, some sporting organisations fear that music is so potent it can give an edge over other competitors, prompting bans when the sport is being performed.

"The most decorated Olympian of all time, Michael Phelps, is particularly well known for his use of a brash and aggressive hip-hop playlist in the competitive arena," says Dr Karageorghis. "He is able to block out the pre-race hullaballoo, focus intently on the task at hand, and reinforce his identity as the imperturbable principal of the pool through his distinctly rap-centric soundtrack."

Yet most people are not harnessing music to its full potential, says Dr Karageorghis, who believes his book is the first to formalise how music can be applied to exercise, be you an athlete or a reluctant gym-goer.

"Music can have a profound effect on our emotional state and every facet of music can contribute towards this," he explains.

Dr Karageorghis also admits that there are cases where music can be detrimental to exercise. The distinction comes down to whether a person has what he describes as an "associative" or "dissociative" attentional style. For instance, gym fanatics and elite athletes who continuously monitor their pace and energy levels in order to achieve optimum performance can find music too distracting. Dissociators, on the other hand, rely on stimulation to divert their attention from the pain.

Dr Karageorghis says music could therefore be used to tackle the obesity epidemic. "We have a huge problem with inactivity, obesity and type 2 diabetes in the Western world, and I am convinced that music and exercise form a large part of the solution. I have this theory that if the NHS were to pay couch potatoes to engage in thrice-weekly exercise-to-music sessions, it would make a huge long-term saving in their budget."

Studies into amateur running clubs, for example, have shown that music prevents joggers from hearing heavy breathing or pounding footsteps of themselves or those around them, which can be demotivating. In this way, suggests Ian Gummery, Course Leader in Sport Psychology and Coaching at London Metropolitan University, other distractions can achieve similar effects to music.

"Thinking of other things such as an upcoming holiday, or even working through a current problem in your mind which may be totally unrelated to sport can achieve the same effect," he says.

Dr Costas Karageorghis chimes that verbal encouragement – like being yelled at by a personal trainer – can also boost performance, as well as finding an exercise buddy with similar goals and fitness level to stoke friendly competition. Still, nothing works quite like music, says Dr Karageorghis – not even downing a double espresso before hitting the treadmill.

So, what is the secret to piecing together the perfect workout playlist? Research suggests that rhythm is the most important factor for the average gym-goer, says Dr Karageorghis, whereas those competing at a professional level are more likely to benefit from music they have a strong emotional connection with.

And if hip-hop is good enough for Michael Phelps, that's a good enough starting point for us.

19 September 2016

⇨ The above information is reprinted with kind permission from *The Independent*. Please visit www.independent.co.uk for further information.

Office workers of England – stand up for your health!

Workers have been warned to "stand up for at least two hours a day in [the] office," according to *The Daily Telegraph*. It says these are the first official health guidelines on the issue.

The guidance comes from a panel of experts, commissioned by Public Health England, which provides recommendations aimed at helping employers know what to aim for when trying to make workplaces less sedentary and more active. They say that this could potentially improve productivity and profitability, for example by reducing sickness.

This guidance has been prompted by a growing body of evidence that sedentary behaviour can increase the risk of a range of chronic diseases such as obesity, type 2 diabetes and high blood pressure. Some experts have gone as far as saying that "sitting is the new smoking".

Dr Ann Hoskins, Deputy Director for Health and Wellbeing, Healthy People, Public Health England said: "This research supports the Chief Medical Officer's recommendations to minimise how much we sit still. Being active is good for your physical and mental health. Simple behaviour changes to break up long periods of sitting can make a huge difference."

Why was the guidance needed?

The aim was to provide employers and staff working in office environments initial guidance on how to combat the potential risks of long periods of seated office work. The authors of the article report that recently more evidence has been published about the links between sedentary behaviour, including at work, and cardiovascular disease, diabetes and some cancers. These conditions are leading causes of ill health and death. As a result, they say that the guidance hopes to support those employers and staff who want to make their working environments less sedentary and more active.

How was the guidance developed?

The experts based their guidance on the available evidence. This included long-term epidemiological studies looking at the effects of sedentary behaviour, and studies of getting workers to stand or move more often.

They ranked the quality of the studies using the American College of Sports Medicine system – this ranks studies from the highest quality grading of A (overwhelming data from randomised controlled trials (RCTs), to D (a consensus judgement from the panel). They based their recommendations on the best available evidence.

They say that the key evidence used in developing their guidance was:

⇨ data from a longer term retrospective national health and fitness survey which found that standing (or having some movement) for more than two hours a day at work was associated with lowering of risks, and those standing for at least four hours had the lowest risks. This was independent of a person's physical activity

⇨ data from a number of observational or short-term interventional studies where there were changes in "cardiometabolic" and ergonomic risk factors (such as energy expenditure, blood glucose, insulin, muscle function and joint sensations), when the total accumulated time spent standing or having some movement was more than two hours a day.

In preparing their recommendations they used other experts as a "sounding board". The guidance was also externally peer reviewed when it was submitted for publication.

What were the recommendations?

The recommendations for workers who are in mainly desk-based occupations, were broadly that:

⇨ The initial aim should be to work towards getting at least two hours a day of standing and light walking during working hours, and eventually work up to a total of four hours per day.

⇨ Seated work should be regularly broken up with standing work and vice versa. Sit–stand adjustable desk stations were highly recommended.

⇨ Similar to avoiding remaining in a static seated position for a long time, remaining in a static standing posture should also be avoided.

⇨ Movement does need to be checked and corrected on a regular basis, especially if a person experiences musculoskeletal sensations. Occupational standing and walking have not been shown to cause low back and neck pain, and can provide relief.

⇨ People new to adopting more standing-based work may have some musculoskeletal sensations and fatigue as part of the process of adapting to this. If these cannot be relieved either by changing posture or walking for a few minutes, then the worker should rest, including sitting, in a posture that relieves the sensations. If discomfort persists, then medical advice should be sought.

⇨ Employers should promote the message to their staff that prolonged sitting, across work and leisure time, may significantly increase one's risk of cardiometabolic diseases and premature death.

The experts acknowledge that more evidence is required to add greater certainty to their recommendations. They call for longer term, prospective and large-scale RCTs to assess standing and light activity interventions in real office environments and their effect on long-term health outcomes. They note that future refinements to their recommendations will be needed as more evidence is published.

2 June 2015

⇨ The above information is reprinted with kind permission from NHS Choices. Please visit www.nhs.uk for further information.

© NHS Choices 2017

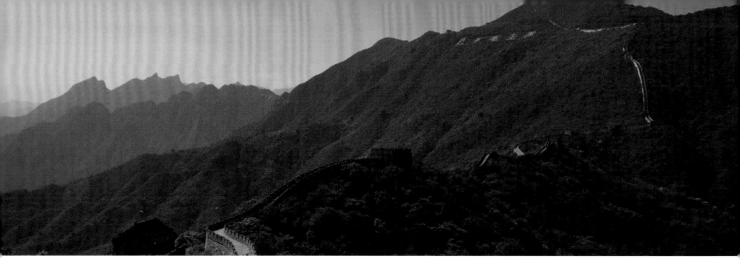

Prescribing exercise outdoors could reduce obesity, say councils

Doctors prescribing exercise outdoors to patients would get more people doing physical activity and help reduce obesity, say councils.

The Local Government Association, which represents more than 370 councils, is calling for a similar model to the 'green prescription' in New Zealand that gets people outdoors, to be introduced in England and Wales.

In New Zealand, where the scheme has been running since 1998, eight out of every ten GPs have issued green prescriptions to patients. These are forwarded to a patient support person who encourages the patient to be more active through phone calls, face-to-face meetings or a support group. Progress is reported back to the GP.

> A new report reveals that the English adult population made around 2.93 billion visits to natural environments between March 2013 to February 2014 – the highest number for 5 years.
>
> In total, 58% of the population claim to make one leisure visit or more to the outdoors every week and between March 2013 to February 2014, it is estimated that the 42.3 million adults resident in England took a total of 2.93 billion visits to the natural environment.
>
> Visiting the natural environment for health or exercise accounted for an estimated 1.3 billion visits to the natural environment between March 2013 to February 2014. Respondents to the survey also agreed that being outdoors made them feel 'calm and relaxed' and the proportion agreeing that a visit was 'refreshing and revitalising' was at its highest in the most recent survey.
>
> *15 January 2015*
>
> *© Crown Copyright*

A recent survey of patients given green prescriptions in the country found 72 per cent noticed positive changes to their health, 67 per cent improved their diet and more than half (51 per cent) felt stronger and fitter.

Rather than just issuing prescriptions for medicines, the LGA says that if GPs in England and Wales wrote down moderate physical activity goals, it would benefit patients who are obese or overweight.

These could be outdoor walks, activities in parks, or family exercise classes run by the local council.

Some GPs are already taking part in schemes to get patients exercising and enjoying the great outdoors, such as in Dartmoor and Exmoor.

Councils, which have responsibility for public health, want to see the measures rolled out nationwide.

The latest guidelines for health professionals say that one in four patients would exercise more if advised to do so by a GP or nurse. Research published in the *British Medical Journal* found that a green prescription can improve a patient's quality of life over 12 months and help people live longer, healthier lives.

Cllr Izzi Seccombe, Chairman of the LGA's Community Wellbeing Board, said:

"Not every visit to a GP is necessarily a medical one. By writing formal prescriptions for exercise, it would encourage people to do more physical activity.

"There are some instances where rather than prescribing a pill, advising on some type of moderate physical activity outdoors could be far more beneficial to the patient.

"This could be going on organised walks, conservation work with a local park group, or gardening at home.

"The green prescription model is something that could help to tackle major health conditions such as obesity and diabetes. There are already some good examples where this is being

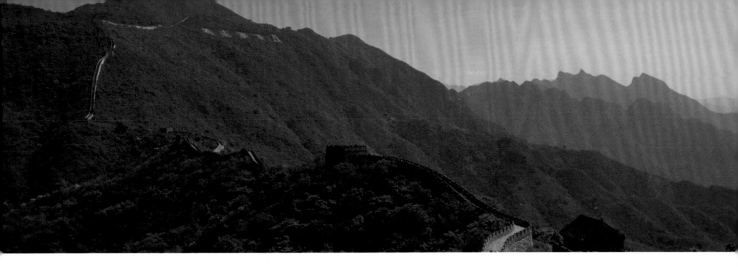

piloted in the UK, and it is something we should consider on a nationwide basis."

Steven Ward, ukactive Executive Director, said: "Britain is in the grip of a cradle to grave physical inactivity crisis and the great outdoors is a fantastic gateway for getting people moving again.

"Physical activity has been hailed as a miracle cure which can help to treat and prevent more than 20 lifestyle-related diseases and if GPs were to prescribe this it would bring huge benefits to people's physical and mental health.

"As ukactive has seen with our targeted intervention programme Let's Get Moving, empowering at-risk patients to take part in regular physical activity transforms lives and offers a potent antidote to our growing health crisis."

Case studies

Dartmoor and Exmoor National Park Authorities

Green prescription-type pilots have been trialled in Devon and Somerset. A three-year scheme is under way where GPs are encouraging patients to visit the national parks as part of their treatment or as an alternative to medication. Surgeries provide Walking for Health Packs to promote walking in the outdoors. If successful, the scheme could be rolled out to national parks elsewhere.

⇨ http://www.somersetlive.co.uk/gps-prescribe-walking-national-parks-instead/story-25260536-detail/story.html

⇨ https://www.gov.uk/government/uploads/system/uploads/attachment_data/file/509916/national-parks-8-point-plan-for-england-2016-to-2020.pdf

⇨ http://www.dartmoor.gov.uk/visiting/accessible-dartmoor/vi-walkingforhealth

Dorset

Weymouth and Portland Borough Council is part of the Natural Choices group which runs activities for GPs to refer patients to. These include walks, conservation work, gardening and sailing. The programme is part of Live Well Dorset, commissioned by Public Health Dorset (https://www.dorsetforyou.gov.uk/natural-choices).

Liverpool

Liverpool City Council and Liverpool Clinical Commissioning Group are delivering a £2.9 million Liverpool Active City Strategy which includes GP referral schemes and activities in parks to tackle obesity and improve people's health and well being (http://www.liverpoolccg.nhs.uk/media/1759/liverpool-active-city-pas-strategy.pdf).

East Riding

East Riding of Yorkshire Council has developed an IT system which connects GPs with leisure centres so they can book patients directly on to an exercise-on-referral scheme. Patients are met by a trainer who is able to tailor a programme to suit the individual (http://www.eastridingleisure.co.uk/goole-leisure-centre/health/live-well/).

Notes to editors

⇨ Just what the doctor ordered. Social prescribing – a guide for local authorities:

· http://www.local.gov.uk/documents/10180/7632544/L16-108+Just+what+the+doctor+ordered+-+social+prescribing+-+a+guide+to+local+authorities/f68612fc-0f86-4d25-aa23-56f4af33671d.

⇨ *British Medical Journal* research on green prescriptions:

· http://www.health.govt.nz/our-work/preventative-health-wellness/physical-activity/green-prescriptions.

⇨ Statistics show that one in four women and one in five men in England are physically inactive, doing less than 30 minutes moderate physical activity a week, and well below the recommended 150 minutes of moderate physical activity a week recommended by the UK Chief Medical Officers.

⇨ Natural England says that for every £1 spent on healthy walking schemes, the NHS could save £7.18 in the cost of treating conditions such as heart disease, stroke and diabetes.

5 September 2016

⇨ The above information is reprinted with kind permission from the Local Government Association. Please visit www.local.gov.uk for further information.

Working together to promote active travel

Shaping the built environment to increase active travel

Because the built environment is associated with how we travel, planners and policymakers have an opportunity to make changes in that environment to promote healthier and more active communities.

It is notable that UK suburbs created in the past 20 to 30 years or so tend to exhibit high levels of car dependence and low levels of active travel, while some of the older or mixed-age neighbourhoods are less car dependent and have high levels of active travel.[1]

Increasing walking and physical activity

Streets and roads make up around three quarters of all public space. Their appearance and the way they function therefore have a significant impact on people's lives. Well-designed, accessible streets can encourage people to walk or cycle more as part of their daily routines, leading to a healthier lifestyle. Streets that encourage people to linger and spend time can also provide economic benefits, for example for local retail.

Local authorities have adopted a range of strategies to increase walking in their neighbourhoods. Evidence on links between walking and the physical environment provide some clear messages for planners. It suggests that people walk more in places with mixed land use (such as retail and housing), higher population densities and highly connected street layouts. These urban forms are associated with between 25% and 100% greater likelihood of walking.[2]

People can also be encouraged to walk more by interventions tailored to their needs, targeted at the most sedentary or at those most motivated to change, and delivered either at the level of the individual or household or through group-based approaches.[3]

Walking can often be combined with public transport, and this can provide a significant boost to physical activity

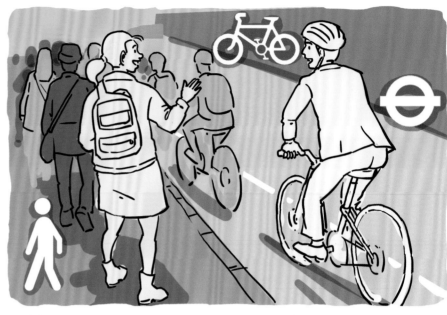

levels[4] while reducing congestion, pollution and road danger. Access to public transport such as buses can be facilitated by providing affordable ticket prices, flexibility in stops, drop-steps to assist getting on and off buses, high-quality travel information, and regular and reliable services.[5]

There is also a growing evidence base on the benefits of 20mph speed limits in support of this[6] and repeated national surveys show strong public support for 20mph in residential streets.[7][8] Many towns and cities in England have either implemented or are committed to 20mph speed limits across much of their road networks.

The *Manual for Streets* changed the Government's approach to the design and provision of residential and other streets. This includes a hierarchy of provision that puts walking and cycling at the top, and following its principles can help design places that encourage active travel.[9]

Increasing cycling

Robust studies have shown that a variety of approaches are associated with increases in cycling. These include:

⇨ an intensive intervention with individuals,

⇨ individualised marketing to households,

⇨ improving infrastructure for cycling, and

⇨ multifaceted town level or city level programmes.[10]

Spatial factors positively associated with cycling include the presence of dedicated cycle routes or paths, separation of cycling from other traffic, high population density, short trip distance, proximity of a cycle path or green space and (for children) projects promoting 'safe routes to school'.[11] PHE and RoSPA have recently published a briefing to help people working in education, public health, school nursing, road safety and others to promote safe active travel to schools.[12]

More generally when considering new developments, how we design our neighbourhoods is key to promoting healthy travel habits, not least in terms of:

⇨ mixed use developments, where local facilities such as shops, GP practices, schools and other services are located, are important in providing short trip distances amenable to routine walking and cycling

⇨ 'filtered permeability' (road design that still allows through-access for walking and cycling, but removes it for motor traffic) to provide direct routes for these modes, which in turn encourages active travel.

Children and neighbourhoods

A key challenge is to enable children to walk or cycle to and from school safely. Action that can encourage this includes developing a school travel plan, providing training and practical support to promote safe cycling, developing walking buses and other partnership work between schools, parents and carers, communities and the local authority.[13]

Some areas have also been experimenting with allowing street closures ('street play') for set periods of time on a regular basis to encourage children to be able to play actively, independently and safely near their own front door. This can help improve children's confidence, self-esteem and resilience as well as encouraging physical activity.[14] An evaluation of play streets in Hackney found that the initiative led to an estimated 8,140 child-hours of outdoor play across 29 streets in a 12-month period. Some 1,600 children were involved.[15]

Older adults and people with disabilities

The built environment is key to maintaining independence and mobility.[16] Factors that can affect older people's physical activity include pedestrian infrastructure, safety, access to amenities and services, aesthetics and environmental conditions.[17] Consultation with people with disabilities has also highlighted the importance of adequate road crossings, pavements, toilets and public seating as well as organisational and attitudinal factors to encourage walking.[18]

It is important to engage people with dementia and their carers in the planning, development and evaluation of the urban realm. For example, having frequent pedestrian crossings with increased crossing times and audible and visual cues are necessary to help people with dementia safely cross the street.[19] Small-scale improvements such as good street lighting or improved road crossings can also encourage movement.[20]

Research suggests a need for constantly maintaining, improving and adapting the pedestrian environment to meet the needs of older people who are likely to be more vulnerable as pedestrians but need the ability to venture outside both for their physical and mental health and wellbeing.

The importance of green spaces

The presence of, and access to, green areas influences physical activity through the whole of the life-course.[21] Access to the natural environment can help increase activity and reduce obesity, with research suggesting that people with good perceived and/or actual access to green space are 24% more likely to be active.[22]

The 2005 *Bristol Quality of Life in your Neighbourhood* survey showed that reported use of green space declined with increasing distance from it. People living closest to the type of green space classified as a 'formal park' were more likely to achieve recommended levels of physical activity and were less likely to be overweight or obese.[23][24]

Rural communities

People living in rural areas and villages may find it as hard to be physically active as people in towns and cities. Difficulties in safely accessing many services by walking, cycling, or by public transport, can pose a real challenge in some rural areas.

A lack of pavements or cycle ways on busy rural roads can discourage use of these travel modes even when moving between towns and settlements not too far apart. A challenge for planners is to consider how access can be improved, and how the needs of walkers and cyclists can be taken into account in the design and planning of the rural road network. The Department of Transport commends adopting a "Safe Systems approach" to build a safer road system,[25] which one local authority has defined as the "need to design a safe environment in which people can move around".[26]

One specific example which promotes physical activity is allowing cycles on buses, so people can get from one town or village to another and then use their bikes to get around at their destination point.

Travel plans

Travel plans[27] are already required for significant new developments such as housing, schools, businesses and healthcare facilities as part of the planning system to demonstrate the impact of such developments on traffic and movement of people.

Public health and transport planners can work together to ensure that such schemes demonstrate how they support shifts from private cars to forms of active travel, and promote the design of safe and attractive neighbourhoods in which people can move around.

Signs of change

There are some signs of change. The total number of miles driven by car has increased, although the average number of car journeys per person in the UK fell by 12% from 1995 to 2013 (with major decreases among young people, men above the age of 30 and London residents). In contrast, the number of female drivers is increasing.

There has been a significant increase in passenger miles using rail transport and the number of cycle journeys has increased in flat, dense urban areas such as London, Cambridge, Oxford and Brighton. Factors behind cycling's popularity within London include significant investment in cycle infrastructure, the introduction of the congestion charge and the introduction of the cycle hire scheme (which has seen annual journeys increase to over ten million in five years).

People of all ages increasingly want to live in walkable, mixed use, public transport-rich communities.[28] There is also evidence that car travel is becoming less popular[29] and that it has become a minority mode of travel for younger commuters.[30]

The challenge now is to roll out good practice across the country.

References

1. Barton H, Horswell M & Millar, P (2012) *Neighbourhood accessibility and active travel, Planning Practice & Research*, 27(2), 117-201.

2. Sinnett, D et al. (2012) *Creating built environments that promote walking and health: A review of international evidence*. Journal of Planning and Architecture 2012: 38.

3. Ogilvie et al. (2007) *Interventions to promote walking: systematic review*. BMJ.9;334(7605):1204.

4. Besser L & Dannenberg A (2006) *Walking to public transit. Steps to help meet physical activity*

recommendations. American Journal of Preventive Medicine, 29(4): 273-280.

5 Broome K, McKenna K, Fleming J & Worrall L (2009) *Bus use and older people: A literature review applying the person-environment-Occupation model in macro practice*. Scandinavian Journal of Occupational Medicine, 16: 3-12.

6 Cairns J, Warren J, Garthwaite K, Greig G & Bambra C (2014) *Go slow: an umbrella review of the effects of 20mph zones and limits on health and health inequalities*. Journal of Public Health, doi:10.1093/pubmed/fdu067.

7 Department of Transport *British Social Attitudes Survey* various years.

8 University of the West of England (2013) *20mph: A survey of GB attitudes and behaviours*. Bristol: UWE.

9 DfT and DCLG (2007) *Manual for Streets*, www.gov.uk/government/publications/manual-for-streets.

10 Yang et al (2010) *Interventions to promote cycling*. BMJ, systematic review. 341:c5293.

11 Fraser S & Lock K (2010) *Cycling for transport and public health: a systematic review of the effect of the environment on cycling*. The European Journal of Public Health, 21, (6), 738-743. (doi:10.1093/eurpub/ckq145).

12 Public Health England & Royal Society for the Prevention of Accidents (2016) *Road injury prevention – resources to support schools to promote safe active travel*. London: PHE.

13 Public Health England & Royal Society for the Prevention of Accidents (2016) *Road injury prevention – resources to support schools to promote safe active travel*. London: PHE.

14 See Play England website: www.playengland.org.uk/our-work/projects/street-play.aspx.

15 Gill, T (2015) *Hackney play streets evaluation report*. Hackney Play Association and Hackney Council.

16 Rosso A, Auchincloss A & Michael Y (2011) *The Urban Built Environment and Mobility in Older Adults: A Comprehensive Review*. Journal of Aging Research, Article ID 816106.

17 Housing Learning and Improvement Network (2016) *Active ageing and the built environment Housing LIN* (in press).

18 Living Streets *Overcoming barriers and identifying opportunities for everyday walking for disabled people* Living Streets (in press).

19 World Health Organisation (2014) *Dementia and age-friendly environments in Europe (AFEE)*. WHO: Copenhagen.

20 Public Health England (2013) *Obesity and the environment*. London: PHE.

21 Institute of Health Equity/Public Health England (2014) *Improving Access to Green Spaces - Health Equity Briefing 8*. Institute of Health Equity. www.gov.uk/government/uploads/system/uploads/attachment_data/file/355792/Briefing8_Green_spaces_health_inequalities.pdf

22 Natural England (2009) *Technical Information Note TIN055: An estimate of the economic and health value and cost effectiveness of the expanded WHI scheme 2009*.

23 Coombes E, Jones A & Hillsdon M. (2010) *The relationship of physical activity and overweight to objectively measured green space accessibility and use*. Social Science & Medicine, Volume 70(6): 816-822.

24 Gong Y, Gallacher J, Palmer S & Fone D (2014) *Neighbourhood green space, physical function and participation in physical activities among elderly men: the Caerphilly Prospective study*. International Journal of Behavioral Nutrition and Physical Activity 2014, 11:40 doi:10.1186/1479-5868-11-40.

25 Department for Transport (2015) *Working together to build a safer road system – British road safety statement*. London: DfT.

26 Bristol City Council (2015) *A Safe Systems Approach to Road Safety in Bristol*.

27 For details see http://planningguidance.communities.gov.uk/blog/guidance/travel-plans-transportassessments-and-statements-in-decision-taking/travel-plans

28 Frontier Group US PIRG Education Fund (2012) *Transportation and the next generation. Why young people are driving less and what it means for transportation policy*.

29 Goodwin P, & Van Dender K (2013) *'Peak Car' – Themes and Issues*. Transport Reviews, 33(3): 243-254.

30 Bristol City Council (2014) *Census Topic Report. Who walks to work?* Bristol City Council.

www.bristol.gov.uk/sites/default/files/documents/council_and_democracy/statistics_and_census_information/2011%20Census%20Topic%20Report%20-%20Who%20walks%20to%20work.pdf accessed 17/02/2015.

May 2016

⇨ The above information is reprinted with kind permission from Public Health England (the Department of Health). Please visit www.gov.uk for further information.

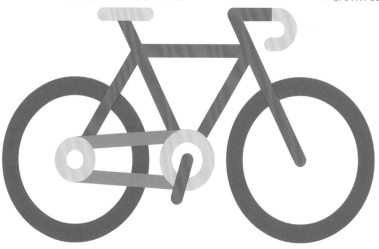

ONLY 9% OF BRITONS CYCLE TO WORK

Ten new "healthy" towns to be built in England

Towns, designed to address problems such as obesity and dementia, will have 76,000 new homes and 170,000 residents.

By Haroon Siddique

Fast food-free zones near schools could soon be a reality in ten NHS England-backed "healthy" new towns designed to encourage people to exercise more, eat better and live independently into old age.

The NHS hopes that by helping to shape the way the towns are built it can begin to address major healthcare problems including obesity and dementia and establish a blueprint that will be followed elsewhere.

The ten towns selected, stretching from Darlington to Devon, will comprise more than 76,000 homes and 170,000 residents. They will be announced formally by the NHS England chief executive, Simon Stevens, at the King's Fund in London on Tuesday.

He said: "The much-needed push to kickstart affordable housing across England creates a golden opportunity for the NHS to help promote health and keep people independent. As these new neighbourhoods and towns are built, we'll kick ourselves if in ten years' time we look back having missed the opportunity to 'design out' the obesogenic environment [which encourage people to eat unhealthily and not take enough exercise], and 'design in' health and well-being.

"We want children to have places where they want to play with friends and can safely walk or cycle to school – rather than just exercising their fingers on video games. We want to see neighbourhoods and adaptable home designs that make it easier for older people to continue to live independently wherever possible. And we want new ways of providing new types of digitally enabled local health services that share physical infrastructure and staff with schools and community groups."

Renowned clinicians, designers and technology experts will work together to help deliver environments that promote healthy lifestyles.

They are likely to include easier access to public transport and safer cycling and pedestrian networks. For instance, there could be so-called dementia-friendly streets, with wider pavements, fewer trip hazards and LCD moving signs, which research suggests people with the disease find easier to navigate.

There will also be an emphasis on workplaces, schools and leisure facilities that encourage physical activity, healthy eating and positive mental health and well-being. Previous attempts to introduce fast food-free zones have been hampered by the legal difficulties of shutting down existing businesses – but this would not be an issue in new towns.

In Darlington, technology will be used to develop a "virtual care home" whereby a group of homes with shared facilities will link directly into a digital care hub to avoid institutionalisation in nursing homes.

Professor Kevin Fenton, the national director for health and well-being at Public Health England, said: "Some of the UK's most pressing health challenges – such as obesity, mental health issues, physical inactivity and the needs of an ageing population – can all be influenced by the quality of our built and natural environment. The considerate design of spaces and places is critical to promote good health. This innovative programme will inform our thinking and planning of everyday environments to improve health for generations to come."

Physical inactivity is a direct factor in one in six deaths, and has an overall economic impact of £7.4 billion. A Design Council guide estimates that a quarter of British adults walk for less than nine minutes a day.

The ten sites, which are at different stages of development, are Whitehill and Bordon in Hampshire; Cranbrook in Devon; Darlington in County Durham; Barking Riverside in London; Whyndyke Farm in Fylde, Lancashire; Halton Lea in Runcorn, Cheshire; Bicester in Oxfordshire; Northstowe in Cambridgeshire; Ebbsfleet Garden City in Kent; and Barton Park in Oxford.

They were chosen from 114 applicants from local authorities, housing associations, NHS organisations and housing developers.

1 March 2016

⇨ The above information is reprinted with kind permission from *The Guardian*. Please visit www.theguardian.com for further information.

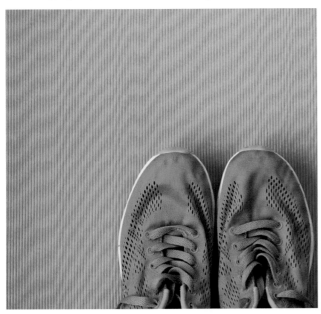

One in three people track health or fitness

Global marketing research firm GfK quizzed 4,900 people in 16 countries, but users in the UK rank well below average.

By Elliot Mulley-Goodbarne

One in three people monitor or track their health and fitness via an online or mobile app, or via a fitness band, clip or smartwatch.

This is according to a survey by global market research firm GfK, which quizzed 4,900 Internet users in 16 countries who currently track their health or fitness.

China leads the way with 45 per cent of the online population monitoring health and fitness in this way, followed by Brazil and the US (29 per cent), Germany (28 per cent) and France (26 per cent).

In the UK, almost a fifth (19 per cent) said that they track their well being using an online service while 16 per cent have previously used online services but do not any more.

The survey also found that 21 per cent of the men and 18 per cent of the women who took the survey in the UK used online apps or gadgets to track their fitness. Those statistics are over ten per cent less than the global average in both respective fields.

When asked why they monitor their health via online app and gadgets, over half said they do so to maintain or improve their fitness condition, with a similar number claiming these apps and gadgets motivated them to exercise. Almost a third said they wanted to lose weight and to have a better night's sleep.

Just eight per cent use health and fitness services to compete with other people.

Broadening appeal

GfK global lead for wearables research Jan Wassmann said: "These findings demonstrate the attraction that health and fitness monitoring has within much wider groups than just the obvious young sports players.

"Manufacturers and retailers can use these insights – combined with our point-of-sales data on purchases of wearable devices – to understand who are their real-life users and why, and tailor their products to deepen that appeal."

7 October 2016

⇨ The above information is reprinted with kind permission from Mobile News. Please visit www.mobilenewscwp.co.uk for further information.

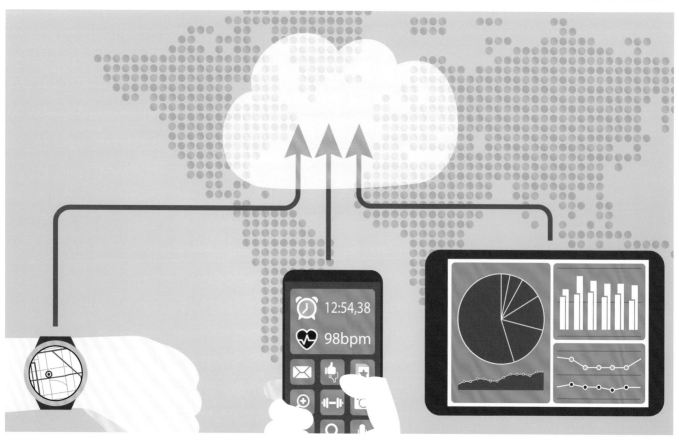

Study blasts fitness trackers' ability to boost health

Work on your willpower instead.

By Natasha Hinde

A study has found that fitness trackers might not benefit health after all.

Researchers discovered that regular use of a fitness tracker or pedometer did not increase activity levels enough to benefit health – even when a financial reward was involved.

It's not the first study to suggest that fitness trackers are not all they're cracked up to be, research published in September found that fitness devices didn't help people lose weight.

A randomised trial involving 800 full-time workers aged 21 to 65 found that, over the course of the year, volunteers who wore activity trackers recorded no change in their step count.

They did, however, moderately increase their amount of aerobic activity by an average of 16 minutes per week.

Cash incentives helped increase exercise levels at six months, but not enough to benefit health. Meanwhile 90% of participants stopped using the devices once incentives stopped.

"We found no evidence that the device promoted weight loss or improved blood pressure or cardiorespiratory fitness, either with or without financial incentives," said lead author Professor Eric Finkelstein from Duke-NUS Medical School in Singapore.

"While there was some progress early on, once the incentives were stopped, volunteers did worse than if the incentives had never been offered, and most stopped wearing the trackers."

Approximately 40% of participants stopped using the activity tracker in the first six months and just 10% were still wearing the tracker at 12 months.

"We saw a large drop off in usage as the study went on. People use these devices for a while, but with time the novelty wears off – this is consistent with how people use trackers in real life," added co-author Professor Robert Sloan from Kagoshima University Graduate School of Medical & Dental Sciences, Japan.

Researchers noted that because people volunteered to participate in the study, they were more likely to be healthy and motivated to be physically active than the average full-time worker.

They said this potentially limits the generalisability of the findings to other groups, but nevertheless the study, which was published in *The Lancet Diabetes & Endocrinology* journal, provides important insights into the use of financial incentives and the health impact of activity trackers.

It's not the first time researchers have examined the impact of fitness trackers and unearthed negative results.

In September, University of Pittsburgh researchers published a study which found trackers were less effective at encouraging people to lose weight than following a diet and exercise plan.

Volunteers who were given fitness armbands lost less weight than those who monitored their own activity.

Scientists believe this is because people become too dependent on gadgets to help them to change their health, resulting in them developing a false sense of security. Instead, they said people should rely on their willpower.

5 October 2016

⇨ The above information is reprinted with kind permission from The Huffington Post UK. Please visit www.huffingtonpost.co.uk for further information.

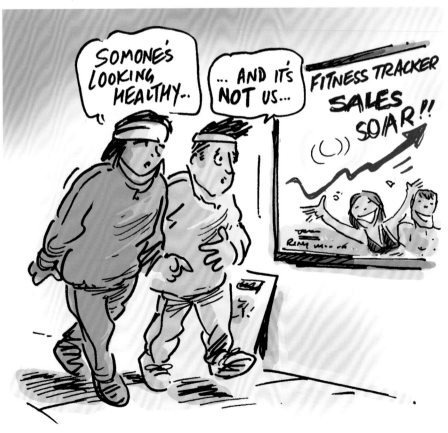

Key facts

⇨ To get all the benefits of exercise, each week adults should aim to do one of the following:

- at least two and a half hours of moderate intensity exercise over a week in bouts of ten minutes or more

- an hour and 15 minutes of vigorous intensity activity

- an equal mix of moderate and vigorous intensity activity

PLUS:

- at least twice-weekly activities that build up muscle strength, such as lifting weights or exercises using your body weight (push-ups and sit-ups for example). (page 1)

⇨ Exercise can reduce your risk of major illnesses, such as heart disease, stroke, type 2 diabetes and cancer by up to 50% and lower your risk of early death by up to 30%. (page 2)

⇨ It's medically proven that people who do regular physical activity have:

- up to a 35% lower risk of coronary heart disease and stroke

- up to a 50% lower risk of type 2 diabetes

- up to a 50% lower risk of colon cancer

- up to a 20% lower risk of breast cancer

- a 30% lower risk of early death

- up to an 83% lower risk of osteoarthritis

- up to a 68% lower risk of hip fracture

- a 30% lower risk of falls (among older adults) (page 2)

⇨ The NHS aerobic activity target is 150 minutes moderate intensity per week (e.g. fast walking/cycling) or 75 minutes vigorous intensity per week (e.g. running, tennis). (page 8)

⇨ 31% of people say that they are aware of the NHS aerobic activity target, but only 40% assert that they met the target over the last three months. 39% are doing less than one session per week. Only one in seven (14%) know about the muscle-strengthening activity target. (page 8)

⇨ Children taking part in organised sports and physical activities at the ages of five, seven and 11 were almost one and a half times more likely to reach a higher than expected level in their Key Stage 2 (KS2) maths test at age 11. No relationship was found between organised sports and activities and KS2 English and science scores. (page 11)

⇨ Levels of physical inactivity in England are very high; nearly 80 per cent of the population do not hit key national government targets. (page 14)

⇨ Nearly everyone (95%) agrees that parks and play areas should be protected from development and 82 per cent feel so strongly that they would be motivated to campaign against a park loss. Two thirds (69%) state that the loss of parks would be detrimental to children's development and half of respondents admitted that they would be less active if their local green space was lost. (page 15)

⇨ Research found almost half of people say using their local park helps them to feel healthier (48%), with 70% of 16- to 24-year-olds also feeling less stressed as a result of having access to green space. Spending quality time with the family and feeling part of a community were also identified as important. Nearly a quarter of people (24%) use their local park at least twice a week. (page 15)

⇨ 14.3 per cent of UK adults now own gym memberships. (page 16)

⇨ Overweight, or pre-obesity, is defined as a BMI of 25–29.9 kg/m2, while a BMI >30 kg/m2 defines obesity. (page 18)

⇨ The average physically active man needs about 2,500 calories a day to maintain a healthy weight, and the average physically active woman needs about 2,000 calories a day. (page 20)

⇨ Between 2005 and 2014, the proportion of adults who were either overweight or obese decreased slightly from 60.9% to 60.5%. However, this is due to a fall in the proportion of overweight adults, as the proportion of obese (I–III) adults has risen from 23.4% to 24.8%. (page 21)

⇨ The UK currently ranks as the country with the highest level of obesity in Europe, with more than one in four (28.1%) adults obese and nearly two out of three (63.4%) overweight. (page 23)

⇨ Today nearly a third of children aged two to 15 are overweight or obese. (page 24)

⇨ 58% of people say they pay a lot of attention to their health, compared to 3% who hardly ever think about it. (page 29)

BMI (body mass index)

An abbreviation which stands for 'body mass index' and is used to determine whether an individual's weight is in proportion to their height. If a person's BMI is below 18.5 they are usually seen as being underweight. If a person has a BMI greater than or equal to 25, they are classed as overweight and a BMI of 30 and over is obese. As BMI is the same for both sexes and adults of all ages, it provides the most useful population-level measure of overweight and obesity. However, it should be considered a rough guide because it may not correspond to the same degree of 'fatness' in different individuals (e.g. a body builder could have a BMI of 30 but would not be obese because his weight would be primarily muscle rather than fat).

Exercise intensity

This refers to how hard you exercise. Exercise intensity can be broken down into light, moderate or vigorous. Light exercise intensity feels easy; you have no noticeable changes in your breathing pattern and don`t break a sweat. Moderate exercise intensity feels somewhat hard; your breath quickens and you develop a sweat after about ten minutes of activity (e.g. leisurely cycling, brisk walk, gardening) Vigorous exercise intensity feels very challenging; you can`t carry on a conversation due to deep, rapid breathing and you develop a sweat after a few minutes of activity (e.g. jumping rope, basketball, running).

Fitness

The condition of being physically healthy (e.g. described as being in shape). Remember, fitness can also apply to our mental health and well-being. A high level of fitness is usually the result of regular exercise and a proper nutrition regime.

Fitness tracker

A wearable device that monitors fitness levels. Many of these devices track steps, heart rate, stairs climbed, sleep patterns, etc.

HIIT (High Intensity Interval Training)

Short bursts of high intensity exercise designed to increase the heart rate. Said to be particularly good for burning fat.

Obesity

When someone is overweight to the extent that their BMI is 30 or above, they are classed as obese. Obesity is increasing in the UK and is associated with a number of health problems, such as an increased risk of heart disease and type 2 diabetes. Worldwide obesity has more than doubled since 1980 and this is most likely due to our more sedentary lifestyle, combined with a lack of physical exercise.

Olympic legacy

This focuses on the idea that the London 2012 Olympics will help to inspire a new generation of aspiring athletes. It also refers to the new facilities that were built to cater for the Olympics, in the hope that they will be used after the Games and continue to grow businesses and help to regenerate the area. For example, the Olympic and Paralympic Village will be converted into thousands of new homes for people to buy and to rent. Visit www.london2012.com to find out more.

Physical activity

Physical activity includes all forms of activity, such as walking or cycling, active play, work-related activity, active recreation such as working out in a gym, dancing, gardening or competitive sport like football. Regular physical activity can reduce the risk of many chronic health conditions including coronary heart disease, type 2 diabetes, cancer and obesity. Regular physical activity also has positive benefits for mental health as it can reduce anxiety and enhance moods and self-esteem, which reduces the risk of depression.

Strength-training

Strength-training activities involve short bursts of effort which results in burning calories whilst building and strengthening muscle. This includes activities such as free weights, weight machines or activities that use your own body weight - such as rock climbing or heavy gardening. The benefits of strength training include increasing bone density, strengthening joints and improving balance, stability and posture. It is recommended that a person should do strength training exercises at least twice a week.

Weight loss surgery

Bariatric (weight-loss) surgery procedures are normally carried out on adults, but in some extreme cases this type of surgery may be considered for children. Weight loss surgery can provide a lasting solution for a wide range of obesity-related problems including diabetes, sleep apnoea and bone or liver disorders. The most common weight loss surgery is a gastric band operation. This is where an elastic band is fitted across the top end of the stomach to restrict the amount of food the person can eat before feeling full. Weight loss surgery is a major medical procedure and shouldn`t be viewed as a quick fix; patients must maintain a strict diet and exercise regime after having the procedure (a person can typically expect to lose between 30 per cent and 50 per cent of their excess body weight). After-care is also important, with the patient having to undergo an intensive treatment programme with a dietician and a psychologist.

Assignments

Brainstorming

⇨ What is fitness?

⇨ How much exercise should you be doing each day, based on your age?

⇨ What is BMI?

⇨ What does the term 'obesity' mean?

Research

⇨ Research how much activity you should be doing per week, based on your age. Create an exercise plan that you believe would be easy to integrate into your daily routine. For example, getting off the bus one stop early and walking the rest of the way, playing sport after school, doing an exercise class or following an exercise DVD at home.

⇨ Research High Intensity Interval Training and create a bullet point list of the pros and cons of this kind of exercise.

⇨ Talk to some friends and relatives about their experiences of PE at school. Think of at least five questions to ask and make a note of the respondent's age and gender. When you have gathered your results, write a summary report no more than two pages long. Include graphs to illustrate the difference between male and female experiences of PE.

⇨ Did you know that half of people in UK cannot run 100 metres? Run 100 metres and time how long it takes you. What level of physical activity do you think you felt while running? Low, moderate or high?

⇨ Research a new sport or fitness activity that you have always wanted to know more about. The more obscure the better! For example, have you ever considered archery or perhaps roller derby? Design a PowerPoint presentation that will persuade people to take-up this unique sport.

Design

⇨ Choose one of the articles from this book and create an illustration that highlights its key message.

⇨ Design a new kind of exercise class aimed at those who are overweight and very nervous about doing group exercise. What kind of exercise could you do to make the class fun and non-intimidating? Work in pairs and create a poster for your class.

⇨ Design a leaflet explaining obesity and its causes.

⇨ Design a poster that will encourage office workers to convert to using standing desks instead of sitting down all day.

⇨ Read the article Ten new "healthy" towns to be built in England on page 37. In pairs, design your own 'healthy town'.

Oral

In pairs, list as many 'moderate intensity' exercises as you can think of that would be easy for a working-mum or dad to fit into their daily routine.

⇨ Choose one of the illustrations from this book and, in pairs, discuss what you think the artist was trying to portray with their image.

⇨ In pairs, create a presentation aimed at people over 60 explaining the benefits of exercise and suggesting ways they can stay active.

⇨ In small groups, discuss why you think 40–54-year-old women are the least likely to meet the NHS exercise guidelines. Share with the rest of your class.

⇨ Do you think it is appropriate for young children to be weighed at school, and for letters to be sent to their parents if they are considered at risk of being overweight? Debate this as a class.

Reading/Writing

⇨ Write a summary of the article How physical activity prevents cancer on page five.

⇨ The article on page 15 says that 'nearly one in five people think their local park or green space [is] under threat of being lost or built on.' Write a letter/formal email to your local MP explaining why your local park is important and the impact it might have on the community's fitness levels if the park were to disappear.

⇨ Imagine you work for a company that manufactures 'wearable technology'. Your company has released a new fitness tracker watch, aimed at young people, and wants to try and sell it in-bulk to local schools. Write a letter to the head teacher of a local school, explaining why you think it would benefit their pupils to wear a fitness tracker and why he/she should invest in them.

Acknowledgements

The publisher is grateful for permission to reproduce the material in this book. While every care has been taken to trace and acknowledge copyright, the publisher tenders its apology for any accidental infringement or where copyright has proved untraceable. The publisher would be pleased to come to a suitable arrangement in any such case with the rightful owner.

Images

All images courtesy of iStock except page 22 from Pixabay and pages 32 & 33 © Tony Bertolino

Icons

Icons on page 17 and 36 were made by Freepik from www.flaticon.com.

Illustrations

Don Hatcher: pages 7 & 28. Simon Kneebone: pages 27 & 39. Angelo Madrid: pages 16 & 34.

Additional acknowledgements

Editorial on behalf of Independence Educational Publishers by Cara Acred.

With thanks to the Independence team: Mary Chapman, Sandra Dennis, Jackie Staines and Jan Sunderland.

Cara Acred

Cambridge, January 2017